New Leads
in Cancer Therapeutics

New Leads
in Cancer Therapeutics

Edited by
Enrico Mihich, M.D.
Director, Department of Experimental Therapeutics and
Grace Cancer Drug Center,
Roswell Park Memorial Institute
Buffalo, New York

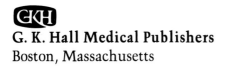

G. K. Hall Medical Publishers
Boston, Massachusetts

G. K. Hall Medical Publishers
70 Lincoln Street
Boston, Massachusetts 02111

81 82 83 84 / 4 3 2 1

Main entry under title:

New leads in cancer therapeutics.

  Bibliography.
  Includes index.
  1. Cancer—Chemotherapy. 2. Antineoplastic agents—
Testing. I. Mihich, Enrico. [DNLM: 1. Neoplasms—
Therapy. QZ266 N532]
RC271.C5N47   616.99'4061   80–17954

ISBN 0–8161–2148–6

Contributors

Ralph J. Bernacki, Ph.D.
Cancer Research Scientist IV, Department of Experimental Therapeutics, Roswell Park Memorial Institute, Buffalo, New York

John S. Bertram, Ph.D.
Cancer Research Scientist V, Department of Experimental Therapeutics, Roswell Park Memorial Institute, Buffalo, New York

Alexander Bloch, Ph.D.
Associate Chief Cancer Research Scientist, Department of Experimental Therapeutics, Roswell Park Memorial Institute, Buffalo, New York

Chi-Hsiung Chang, Ph.D.,
Research Affiliate, Department of Experimental Therapeutics, Roswell Park Memorial Institute, Buffalo, New York

Yung-Chi Cheng, Ph.D.,
University of North Carolina Medical School, Department of Pharmacology, Chapel Hill, North Carolina

Patrick J. Creaven, M.B.B.S., Ph.D.
Chief, Department of Clinical Pharmacology and Therapeutics, Roswell Park Memorial Institute, Buffalo, New York

Lynn Danhauser
Research Affiliate, Department of Experimental Therapeutics, Roswell Park Memorial Institute, Buffalo, New York

Gerald B. Grindey, Ph.D.
Cancer Research Scientist V, Department of Experimental Therapeutics, Roswell Park Memorial Institute, Buffalo, New York

Debora Kramer
Research Affiliate, Department of Experimental Therapeutics, Roswell Park Memorial Institute, Buffalo, New York

Elihu Ledezma, M.D.
Clinician I, Department of Surgical Oncology, Roswell Park Memorial Institute, Buffalo, New York

Enrico Mihich, M.D., Editor
Director, Department of Experimental Therapeutics and Grace Cancer Drug Center, Roswell Park Memorial Institute, Buffalo, New York

Fredika Mikles-Robertson, Ph.D.
Postdoctoral Fellow, University of Southern California Medical Center, Los Angeles, California

Arnold Mittelman, M.D.
Program Director, Colon and Rectal Service, Department of Surgical Oncology, Roswell Park Memorial Institute, Buffalo, New York

Michael J. Morin, Ph.D.
Research Affiliate, Department of Experimental Therapeutics, Roswell Park Memorial Institute, Buffalo, New York

Carl W. Porter, Ph.D.
Cancer Research Scientist IV, Department of Experimental Therapeutics, Roswell Park Memorial Institute, Buffalo, New York

Harvey Preisler, M.D.
Deputy Chief of Medical Oncology, Department of Medical Oncology, Roswell Park Memorial Institute, Buffalo, New York

Fred Rosen, Ph.D.
Associate Chief Cancer Research Scientist, Department of Experimental Therapeutics, Roswell Park Memorial Institute, Buffalo, New York

Youcef M. Rustum, Ph.D.
Cancer Research Scientist V, Departments of Experimental Therapeutics and Clinical Pharmacology and Therapeutics, Roswell Park Memorial Institute, Buffalo, New York

Contents

Acknowledgments

Chapter 2

The authors would like to acknowledge the excellent technical assistance of C. Wrzosek, R. Ghosh, G. Wang, E. Kelly, and N. Riles.

This research was supported in part by U.S. Public Health Service Grant CA-18420, CA-21071, and CA-5834 from the National Cancer Institute, National Institutes of Health, USPHS.

Chapter 3

This investigation was supported in part by Project Grant CA-17156 from the National Institutes of Health, USPHS.

Chapter 5

This contribution is also based on a lecture delivered at the Gordon Conference on "Chemotherapy of Experimental and Clinical Cancer," Meriden, New Hampshire, July 1978.

Chapter 6

Yung-chi Cheng is a scholar of the Leukemia Association of America. This work was supported by Grant CA-18499 from the National Cancer Institute, National Institutes of Health, USPHS.

Chapter 7

This work was supported in part by Public Health Service Grants CA-15757, CA-19814, and CA-13038 from the National Cancer Institute, National Institutes of Health, USPHS.

We acknowledge the valuable contributions of Dr. Y. Rustum, Dr. W. Korytnyk, Dr. W. Klohs, Ms. N. Porter, Mr. J. Froehlich, and Mr. E. Kelly to this study.

Chapter 8
This work was supported by Grant CA-21359 from the National Cancer Institute, National Institutes of Health, USPHS.

Chapter 9
Throughout the course of these studies the authors have had the benefit of skilled technical assistance provided by Ms. L. Caballes, Ms. N. Kaars, Ms. B. Ganis, Mr. J. Miller, and Ms. D. Ogden. The investigation was supported by Grants CA-22153 and CA-13038 from the National Cancer Institute, National Institutes of Health, USPHS. The impetus for the studies involving MGBG was provided by Dr. Chandrakant Dave, who died January 10, 1978. The authors are extremely grateful for his encouragement in this project, and also to Dr. S. N. Pathak for her early contributions to this study.

Introduction

Enrico Mihich, M.D.

Considerable progress in cancer therapeutics has been achieved since the mid-forties, when the initial trials of antifolates, steroids, and alkylating agents marked the beginning of cancer chemotherapy as we know it today. Advances have increased the options available in treating the patient with a specific tumor type or with a tumor at a specific stage, as well as in terms of the types of cancer for which effective treatments can be instituted.

Despite obvious advances, particularly in the treatment of leukemias, lymphomas, Hodgkin's disease, certain types of choriocarcinoma, Wilms's tumor, and certain skin tumors, many limitations must be overcome before chemotherapy by itself can be widely and generally used as the primary treatment in the management of the solid tumors. The primary limitation is that most of the anticancer drugs developed to date are also toxic to normal tissues and have limited selectivity for the tumors they are meant to treat. Consequently, in many cases even a limited degree of natural or acquired resistance to a drug cannot be overcome without incurring unacceptable toxicity. Attempts to overcome these limitations and to further improve the effectiveness of cancer therapeutics should focus on multiple approaches.

The development of new drugs with improved selectivity of action against tumor cells is a primary goal based on 1) acquisition of new information about the biological and biochemical characteristics of cancer cells that may result in new types of drugs affecting these cells through selective action upon newly identified targets; 2) development of analogs of known active agents that have more favorable pharmacological characteristics than their parent compounds and, consequently, improved selectivity of antitumor action; 3) careful study of new chemical structures that derive from semiempirical or even empirical approaches in screening; and 4) the development of agents and treatments that act against tumors indirectly by augmenting the physiological responses of the host against the tumor or by mimicking these responses.

Clarification of the biochemical and pharmacological basis of the selective toxicity of known drugs and treatments is another important goal, since in many cases available agents may not be used under conditions that maximize selectivity of antitumor action or are not used against tumors which may be unrecognized targets of their action. Improvements in the clinical utilization of the well-known antimetabolite methotrexate during the past 30 years provides a convincing example of the opportunities open to the chemotherapist for identifying new target tumors and designing new regimens with increased therapeutic advantages.

The clinical development of chemotherapeutic regimens utilizing known active drugs in multiple combinations received major impulse in the 1960s and has radically changed the outlook on cancer chemotherapy by demonstrating the [possibility of inducing] long-term survival without detectable disease. The development of new combination chemotherapeutic regimens represents a continuing effort and has the potential for additional significant improvements based on novel approaches. Indeed, as more knowledge is acquired on the determinants of the selectivity of action of known drugs, opportunities increase to develop new combination therapies. These can be based not only on synergisms among active agents, but also on such mechanisms as the potentiation of active agents by compounds affecting their rate of activation or inactivation, or their potentiation by compounds augmenting the response of target tumor cells through a favorable modification of the biochemical and pharmacological determinants of their action.

While chemotherapy has become recognized as an effective modality in the management of certain types of cancer, it is apparent that additional therapeutic advantages may be achieved through its combination with other treatment modalities. Increased attention is being given to chemotherapy as a potentially curative adjunct to presumed radical surgery and radiotherapeutic treatments. Moreover, the possibility is being explored that modifiers of biological responses of the host against the tumor may provide an effective and probably relatively nontoxic means to eliminate residual tumor cells after cytoreductive treatment with antiproliferative or cytocidal chemotherapy is given alone or in combination with radiotherapy or surgery. If judiciously applied, this multimodality approach in cancer therapeutics may turn out to be at least as profitable as the systematic introduction of combination chemotherapy was in the 1960s.

The approaches already mentioned are all directed toward the improved elimination of tumor cells in patients with a given clinically defined tumor type. Increased attention is also being given to the possibility that chemotherapy may be designed for the individual patient, based on the identification of his or her key pharmacological and biochemical determinants of drug action. Initial steps are being taken in this direction particularly with certain antimetabolites and the anthracyclines, and the results obtained to date seem to encourage further efforts in this difficult area of clinical biochemical pharmacology.

Several of the approaches mentioned here are being pursued in the Department of Experimental Therapeutics and the Grace Cancer Drug Center of Roswell Park Memorial Institute, in cooperation with the Institute's clinical departments. Some of the directions pursued were selected as representative and discussed during a one-day seminar held in the fall of 1978 as part of the Institute's continuing medical education program. Updated versions of these presentations are the subject of this volume.

The topics discussed include 1) the basic process of developing new drugs for clinical use, with acquisition of maximal information and consequent optimal evaluation in human beings; 2) the study of the pharmacological and biochemical determinants of antimetabolite action in individual patients as a prerequisite for the potential design of individualized chemotherapy; 3) the design of novel therapies with antifolates, based on the augmentation of antitumor effectiveness, with decreased toxicity as an example of the therapeutic modulation of antimetabolite action by metabolites; 4) the role that steroid receptors and their regulation might have in determining responsiveness of tumors to hormones and related agents; 5) the basis for the development of new nucleosides as a family of compounds with potential antitumor activity; 6) the biochemical basis for the design of new compounds and treatments selectively affecting deoxynucleotide metabolism in tumor cells; 7) the possible advantages offered by the plasma membrane of cancer cells as a site for therapeutic intervention; 8) new ideas stemming from studies of cell-to-cell contact and growth control in cell populations that may lead to the design of new types of treatments; and 9) the opportunities offered by electron microscopy in identifying ultrastructural changes in cells affected by drugs and in providing insights leading to the design of new treatments. The emphasis in this volume is on providing a few examples of the kinds of approaches that are being pursued to provide new leads toward the development of improved cancer chemotherapy.

Chapter 1

Preclinical and Clinical Pharmacology in Drug Development

Patrick J. Creaven, M.B.B.S., Ph.D. and Enrico Mihich, M.D.

The emphasis in this book is, rightly, on novel approaches to cancer treatment in both the development of new therapies and the development of ways in which established drugs and therapies can be used more effectively. It must be recognized, however, that much of the advance in the drug treatment of cancer over the past 30 years has come from the introduction of new antineoplastic agents, and there remains an acute need for the development of drugs which are more effective, more selective, and less toxic than those currently available. This chapter will deal with some aspects of the development of new agents, with particular reference to the role which preclinical and clinical pharmacology can play in this process, and with specific emphasis on the program of drug development of the Grace Cancer Drug Center, the drug development arm of Roswell Park Memorial Institute. We shall first attempt to summarize the broad general principles of new drug development and then give three examples of current studies with antineoplastic agents under development in the Grace Cancer Drug Center.

Discovery of New Drugs

Development of new anticancer drugs starts with the demonstration of antitumor activity. Some of the approaches that have been used for the discovery of new antineoplastic agents are listed here:
1. Random screening
2. Screening of compounds from specific sources (e.g., fermentation broths)

3. Synthesis and testing of analogs of known antineoplastic agents
4. Rational synthesis employing biochemical principles or other scientific rationales
5. Serendipity

Random Screening

Random screening has been an accepted method for searching for new antineoplastic agents since the establishment of the Cancer Chemotherapy National Service Center (CCNSC) in the mid-fifties. Since that time, the CCNSC and its successors have been responsible for the screening of approximately 15,000 compounds a year from diverse sources (1). As a method of identifying new agents, screening is a procedure with low yield and high cost, and for this reason it is currently undergoing some reevaluation. Its potential advantage is that it has the capability of identifying totally novel structures which could interfere with as yet unrecognized mechanisms for cell growth peculiar to tumor cells, thus providing us with the long-awaited non-cytotoxic antitumor agent. So far this has not occurred, and the number of compounds currently used for the clinical treatment of cancer whose antitumor activity was identified by purely random screening is relatively small. It seems reasonable to predict that random screening will become relatively less important in the overall program for the identification of antitumor agents in the future (2).

Screening Compounds From Specific Sources

The screening of compounds from specific sources is more efficient than random screening. For example, a number of clinically active antitumor agents including daunorubicin, adriamycin, bleomycin, streptonigrin, mitomycin-C, and mithramycin are all derived from different species of Streptomyces. Screening of products isolated from members of this genus would, therefore, be potentially much more fruitful than random screening as the starting point for an attempt to isolate new antitumor agents.

Analog Development

Analogs constitute another high-yield source of new active agents. Once a compound has proved to have clinical activity against tumors, it is customary to attempt to develop analogs designed either to increase antitumor efficacy or to decrease or eliminate unwanted features of the compound such as specific target organ toxicities. An analog may turn out to have a somewhat different spectrum of antitumor activity or toxicity than the parent compound. This may be an advantage, as happened in the case of adriamycin, an analog of daunorubicin whose antitumor spectrum for solid tumors is broader than that of the parent compound.

Rational Synthesis

Many of the antimetabolites in current use are antitumor agents of rational chemical design, although, as in the case of cytosine arabinoside (ara-C), the original rationale may prove to be erroneous. Because it differs from cytidine in the stereochemistry of the 2-position of the sugar, and because this position is the site of reduction of ribose to deoxyribose, it was felt that ara-C would be an effective inhibitor of the reduction step of deoxyribonucleotide biosynthesis (3), whereas it was found that the compound acts by inhibiting DNA polymerase (4). Cyclophosphamide is an example of a rationally synthesized alkylating agent precursor that turned out to be effective for the "wrong" reasons. Designed as a pro-drug which would release nor-nitrogen mustard inside the tumor cell (5), it was found to be activated in the liver without giving rise to substantial amounts of nor-nitrogen mustard (6, 7).

Since compounds developed by rational chemical design are among the compounds most likely to have antitumor efficacy, their development is a logical and relatively economical approach and is the one being pursued in the Grace Cancer Drug Center.

Serendipity

Serendipitous discovery of a compound's antitumor activity is of importance because it may, as in the case of cis-diamminedichloroplatinum-II (cisplatin), lead to a new class of antitumor agents (8) that can then form the starting point for analog development.

Stages of Preclinical Drug Development

Table 1.1 lists the stages in preclinical drug development. Listed in the left column are those procedures which form part of a routine drug development program. On the right are a series of procedures which, while not strictly required in order to introduce an antitumor drug into the clinic, are of considerable importance and should be included as part of the regular development of all drugs. Although it is not essential to perform in vitro tests of antitumor activity (essentially tests of cytotoxicity), in vitro tests are normally included for economic reasons, since large numbers of compounds can undergo initial screening relatively cheaply by this means. The Grace Cancer Drug Center approach to the identification of antitumor activity in vitro and in vivo will be discussed briefly later in this chapter.

Table 1.1   Stages in Preclinical Drug Development

Required Procedures	Desirable Procedures
Identification of antitumor activity in vitro	Preclinical pharmacokinetics and metabolism studies
Identification of antitumor activity in vivo	Mode of action studies
Preclinical toxicology	Drug combination studies
Formulation	
Carcinogenicity testing	
Mutagenicity testing	

Preclinical Toxicology

Table 1.2 analyzes the purposes and uses of preclinical toxicology. As can be seen from the table, a major purpose of preclinical toxicology is to predict for the characteristics of the toxicity which will be seen when a drug is used clinically. The reliability and efficiency of preclinical toxicology have recently been reviewed in detail (9, 10) and will not be discussed extensively here. Suffice it to say that animal systems are able to predict with reasonable efficiency the dose-limiting toxicity to rapidly proliferating tissues, which is the characteristic toxicity of most of the antitumor agents, and can also effectively predict toxicity to the liver, kidney, and lung, although in these cases with a larger number of false-positive results. Toxicological tests in animals do not adequately predict toxicity that appears only after prolonged dosage or toxicity in some other human organ systems including organs of special sense. In addition, while testing in several animal species is useful for the overall quantitative prediction of toxicity, the use of data from the mouse should be given greater emphasis than is usual in evaluating toxicity data.

Formulation

The development of a usable formulation is clearly a prerequisite for putting any drug into clinical trial. Requirements for successful formulation include solubility, stability, and sterility. Problems in developing a successful formulation are perhaps more acute with antitumor agents than with other classes of drugs, both because as a class they have a greater tendency than other drugs to be unstable and because intravenous (and therefore soluble) formulations are generally preferred for antitumor agents. Sometimes, as in the case of 5-azacytidine, it is not possible to

Table 1.2   Preclinical Toxicology

Species:	Mice	Rats	Dogs
Purposes:	1) To exclude unacceptable drugs		
	2) To predict for toxicity characteristics in human beings		
Used to Predict:	1) Quantitative toxicity		
	2) Qualitative toxicity		
	3) Kinetics of toxicity		
	4) Reliability of toxicity		
	5) Reversibility of toxicity		
	6) Steepness of the dose response curve		

make a formulation which is stable for prolonged periods, so the infusion solution must be changed at intervals. Sometimes solubility problems are such that a complex mixture of solubilizers must be used, as in the case of the epipodophyllotoxins VM26 and VP16.

Carcinogenicity and Mutagenicity Tests

Table 1.1 lists carcinogenicity and mutagenicity tests as normally required. Neither of these tests is strictly required for antitumor agents at present, but there is likely to be increasing pressure to make them mandatory. Many antitumor agents, particularly alkylating agents, are strongly carcinogenic and mutagenic. This was not a problem while antitumor agents were relatively ineffective because patients did not survive long enough to experience the carcinogenic effects, and most patients with advanced cancer were either unable to become pregnant or chose not to do so. With the increase in long-term survival of patients with certain types of tumors, the development of second, probably iatrogenic, malignancies has become more frequent. Mutagenicity is much less of a problem, as patients treated with intensive long-term chemotherapy tend to be sterile, but increasing awareness of the potential of drugs to produce fetal malformations may result in more mutagenic testing of antitumor agents.

Pharmacokinetic and Metabolism Studies

Studies of pharmacokinetics, drug metabolism, mode of action, or drug combinations are not required before an antineoplastic drug undergoes clinical trial. There is, however, a developing and increasing consensus that such studies, particularly preclinical pharmacokinetic and drug metabolism studies, are of major importance and should become an integral part of preclinical antitumor drug development. These preclinical studies are already part of the preclinical development of non-antineoplastic agents.

The primary purpose of pharmacokinetic studies is to develop information on the pharmacokinetics of a drug in animals, information that can then be used to help in the design and monitoring of the agent's initial trial in human beings. Such information can, however, also be used in evaluating the toxicity and antitumor efficacy data of the drug in animals, particularly data on schedule dependency. Moreover, if it is found that there are large quantitative differences between toxicity in humans and in animals, it may be possible to explain these differences by comparing human and animal pharmacokinetics. Knowledge of pharmacokinetics may also alert the clinician to the possibility of increased drug toxicity in relation to organ malfunction, specifically renal or hepatic disease. An outline of these studies is given below:

To define the kinetics of absorption, distribution, metabolism, and excretion

1. Absorption: For drugs given orally, rate and completeness of absorption and factors affecting the absorption
2. Distribution: Rapidity of diffusion from the vascular space; volume of distribution
3. Metabolism: Rate of metabolism ⎱ Rate of
4. Excretion: Rate of appearance in urine ⎰ plasma decay
5. Purpose: To predict for human pharmacokinetics, to guide design of clinical trials, to develop information on species differences, to attempt to correlate with toxicity, and to attempt to correlate with response

Mode of Action and Drug Combination Studies

Mode of action studies and drug combination studies can be considered together because, conceptually, knowledge of the mode of action of the drug can be used for rational drug combination, although this is not always the way in which drug combinations have been developed clinically in the past. For example, knowledge of the locus of inhibition of the metabolic pathway by an antimetabolite can lead to the rational use of either sequential blockade of this pathway or blockade of parallel pathways to add to the effect of the original drug (11). Another way in which knowledge of mode of action can be successfully used clinically is in use of the appropriate salvage metabolites to modulate the toxicity and, it is hoped, the antitumor efficacy of an agent (11), as has recently been done with thymidine used in combination with methotrexate (12, 13) and 5-fluorouracil (FU) (14). Although mode of action and drug combination studies are or should be an integral part of any drug development program, they need not be performed before clinical drug use. Such studies are often difficult to carry out, take many years, and can be performed along with the initial clinical trial of the agent. However, the availability of information of this sort by the time the drug has reached the appropriate stage of clinical development, which could be used either to enhance the antitumor efficacy, modulate toxicity, or possibly in the future to turn an antitumor agent with only marginal efficacy by itself into one of high effectiveness would not only be a distinct gain but might give a useful clinical role to agents that would otherwise have to be discarded.

Clinical Trial

Once a drug has been found to have the necessary efficacy in experimental animals, has shown itself to be sufficiently free from insurmountable toxicological problems, and once an appropriate formulation is available, the drug will proceed to clinical trial, which is carried out in a series of phases. These phases are listed in table 1.3, which also lists the pharmacological studies that are appropriately run concurrently with the clinical studies. The purpose of clinical and pharmacological studies is not only to gain increased information about the drug, permitting its more efficacious and less hazardous use in clinical practice, but to generate information for the development of analogs with greater effectiveness or less toxicity, or both, or for development of ways in which the toxicity can be modulated as has just been mentioned. It should be clear that pharmacological and human toxicological studies cannot be performed once and for all, but must be ongoing evaluations of the drug in clinical use. This is a particularly important consideration for toxicities that occur only after prolonged use of the drug or that occur very sporadically. As has been mentioned and previously noted (9, 15), these toxicities are unlikely to be predicted from animal studies and will become evident only after careful observation of the drug in clinical use, usually in well-controlled clinical settings.

The phases of clinical drug evaluation listed in table 1.3 are initial evaluation of toxicity in human beings and initial therapeutic effectiveness (Phase I); demonstration that the drugs do indeed have significant antitumor efficacy against a variety of tumors in human beings (Phase II); and testing of the efficacious drugs against standard agents or therapies currently used to treat the same disease, in a well-designed, controlled study (Phase III). Testing to establish the superiority of the new over the old should apply not only to new drugs but also to new treatment modalities and therapies. The failure to do this in a convincing fashion has left us, for example, many years after the introduction of high-dose and very high-dose methotrexate, without a convincing demonstration that

Table 1.3   Stages in Clinical Drug Development

Studies of Toxicity and Therapeutic Efficacy	Appropriate Concurrent Pharmacological Studies
1. Human toxicology and initial therapeutic evaluation (Phase I)	Clinical pharmacology
2. Human antitumor efficacy (Phase II)	Clinical pharmacology in disease states
3. Clinical usefulness (Phase III)	Parameters of response
4. Use in combinations and combined modalities	Drug interactions
5. Use in the adjuvant setting	Pharmacology and toxicology of long-term use

this treatment modality is markedly superior to methotrexate given in the conventional way. In such trials, of course, it is not necessary for the drug to show increased therapeutic efficacy if it can demonstrate superiority by reason of, for example, diminished toxicity, greater patient acceptance, greater ease of adminstration, lack of cross-resistance with useful agents, or difference in toxicity spectrum to facilitate use in combination. As more effective agents come into clinical use, however, it becomes more difficult for new agents to become established, especially as the agents already in use have had their optimal mode of use worked out. The new agent will often be tested on the schedule that has been used for the older agent, a schedule which may not be optimal for the competitor. This may at times lead to discouragement on the part of those responsible for new drug development. It is important to realize, however, that in this activity the chances of success are small, but the rewards for success for the patient are large.

Initial Clinical Trial (Phase I)

The objectives of the initial clinical trial (Phase I) are to define, in the minimum number of patients and in the minimum time compatible with patient safety:

1. The maximum tolerated dose, generally on at least two schedules of administration
2. The dose-limiting and other characteristic toxicities
3. The kinetics, reversibility, and interpatient variability of the toxic manifestations
4. The steepness of the dose response curve

5. The absence of any qualitatively prohibitive toxicity which would preclude further study of the compound

The initial clinical trial is the groundwork for a full therapeutic trial using the schedule or schedules determined in the Phase I trial.

Before a compound can be placed into clinical trial, a decision must be made on the following critical factors:

1. Starting dose and route
2. Starting schedule (often more than one)
3. Dose escalation
4. Entry requirements
5. Observations to be made and their frequency
6. Number of patients to be entered at each dose level
7. Whether to escalate in the same patient
8. Length of the observation period

The approach to decisions regarding these factors has recently been discussed in detail (9, 10) and will only be outlined here.

The starting dose should be determined after consideration of all of the information available at the time the drug enters clinical trial, including 1) the toxic dose in the animal species tested; 2) the steepness of the drug's dose response curve; 3) the variability of response within animal species and between animal species; 4) the pharmacokinetics in animals, including the variability of the pharmacokinetics and drug metabolism from species to species; and 5) the characteristics of analogs that have already been tested clinically.

Similarly, the starting schedule should be determined after consideration of the schedule dependency of antitumor efficacy and toxicity, the pharmacokinetics, and the mode of action of the drug.

Escalation has traditionally been by a series of decremental steps. As has been pointed out, however (9, 10), this procedure is probably not valuable while the drug shows no toxicity, and it is likely that an approach in which the dose is doubled until some biological effect is seen will become more generally used.

Entry requirements will normally include a requirement that a patient's hepatic and renal function be normal so that baseline data on clinical pharmacology and initial clinical toxicology can be obtained.

Clinical Pharmacological Studies

The objectives of clinical pharmacological studies, carried out concomitantly with the Phase I study, are

1. To define the major human pharmacokinetic parameters
2. To study the effect of disease states on the human pharmacokinetic parameters

3. To study drug distribution to specific sites of importance (e.g., tumor, cerebrospinal fluid [CSF])
4. To identify parameters which correlate with toxicity
5. To identify parameters which correlate with response

The major pharmacokinetic parameters that should be determined are the same as those given for preclinical pharmacokinetics. Sufficient data should be obtained on the pharmacokinetics of a drug to enable predictions to be made about the effect of changes in dosage and in schedule of administration on plasma levels and therefore on toxicity, and, presumably, also on efficacy. Information can be gained about specific situations in which the drug might be particularly valuable, for example, information on penetration of a drug into the CSF, indicating that it might be valuable in the treatment of meningeal leukemia. Such information would clearly contribute to optimum use of the drug.

The question whether pharmacokinetic parameters can, in addition, make a contribution to the overall prediction of antitumor response is one of considerable theoretical importance. A major limitation of cancer chemotherapy is the inability of the clinician to predict, particularly with regard to the less responsive solid tumors, which patients will respond to a particular agent. Some progress has been made in this area with breast carcinoma, particularly in relation to estrogen receptor studies, but for most solid tumors we have little information about what determines response to chemotherapeutic agents. We have recently discussed in detail the question of whether pharmacokinetic parameters could potentially be useful to predict response to antitumor agents and concluded that pharmocokinetic parameters alone are unlikely to predict a patient's response to drugs when the dosage, route, and schedule of administration are optimized, but taken together with other parameters of response such as pharmacodynamic and biochemical parameters, pharmacokinetic parameters might contribute to overall response prediction. This is an area in which the information available is extremely sparse, but which is receiving intensive study (16).

Drug Screening in the Grace Cancer Drug Center

The first part of this chapter has served as a brief introduction to the approach to drug development in the Grace Cancer Drug Center at Roswell Park Memorial Institute. Drug screening in the center is normally carried out on compounds that have been synthesized specifically as potential antitumor agents. Therefore, a more elaborate screening to attempt to identify antitumor efficacy is justified than could normally be carried out in a random screen. One approach currently in use and one that undergoes periodic revision is outlined in figure 1.1. The advantage of the

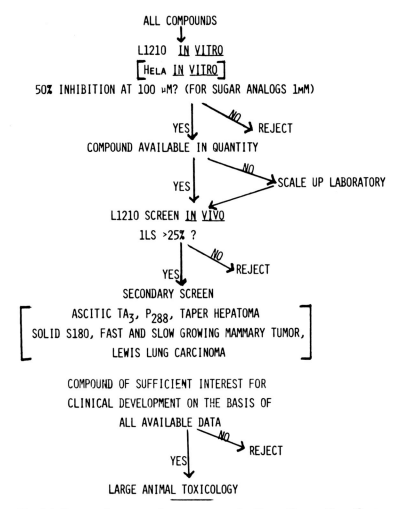

Fig. 1.1 Current drug screening program at the Grace Cancer Drug Center

cascade screen approach is that relatively nonstringent requirements can be used for accepting compounds for further testing. The compounds can then be evaluated in a battery of secondary tests and the decision as to whether they should be developed for clinical trials can be made on an evaluation of all the factors concerned. This approach eliminates the difficulty inherent in relying on a single screening procedure for deciding whether compounds should proceed to clinical trial, namely that if the acceptance criteria are too low, too many compounds will be admitted to the clinic, and if they are high, there is the danger of rejecting potentially useful compounds.

The general approach to toxicological testing in the Grace Cancer Drug Center is outlined here.

A. Lethal doses in three species
B. Course of Intoxication
   1. Gross symptoms
   2. Hematology
   3. Organ function tests
C. Correlation of course of intoxication with
   1. Pathology and histopathology
   2. Pharmacokinetics and biotransformation
D. Recovery from course of intoxication

Newer Approaches to Drug Screening

Drug screening is constantly undergoing reevaluation in the Grace Cancer Drug Center and elsewhere in a continuing effort to improve the predictive ability of screening to identify active and eliminate inactive compounds. Two new approaches that use human tumors in an attempt to predict human tumor response more reliably will be discussed here: the use of human tumor heterotransplants in the nude mouse, and the use of human tumor cells grown in soft agar.

The nude mouse, a hairless mutant homozygous for an autosomal recessive gene that determines congenital absence of the thymus, will receive human tumor heterotransplants that grow but rarely metastasize (17–20). Human tumor lines can be maintained in the nude mouse and used as screens for antitumor agents (21). It must not be assumed, however, that such models will be more predictive of tumor response in patients than animal tumor models; the former must be validated in the same way as the latter. There is, however, another way in which the nude mouse could be used for screening of compounds for antitumor efficacy. A series of tumors of a specific histologic type removed from patients and implanted in the nude mouse could be evaluated for response with a new agent. In this way, an actual response rate of that histologic type of human tumor to the new agent could be obtained. This response rate could then be compared with the actual response rate obtained with the agent in clinical trials. If the heterotransplanted tumor turned out to be a valid predictor of the human tumor response rate for compounds belonging to different classes of agent, this could form a powerful predictive system for evaluating new compounds without the necessity of evaluating them in a wide variety of human tumor types in the clinic. It is clear, however, that while the tumor is a human tumor, the drug delivery system is that of the mouse, and the pharmacokinetic and drug metabolism factors which may modulate antitumor efficacy will be those of the host animal. Target organs for toxicity would also be those of the host animal and not of the patient. These considerations, and the difficulty of maintaining large numbers of nude mice because of their susceptibility to disease, may limit large-scale applications of some of these approaches.

The other new approach is that of growing human tumor cells in soft agar culture systems originally developed for growing murine myeloma (22) and adapted to human tumor cells by Hamburger and Salmon (23, 24). This approach has been extremely successful in the prediction of the resistance of human tumors to antitumor agents, but less successful, although still very impressive, as a predictor of human tumor sensitivity in patients. Human tumor cells grown in soft agar systems are already being used to evaluate new antitumor agents (25, 26). Although this test is a cytotoxicity assay that does not take into account pharmacokinetic factors, should it prove successful for new drug evaluation it would offer the possibility of a dramatic advance in the rapid screening of antitumor agents against a variety of human tumor types. The amount of tumor required is small (generally less than a million cells) and although the cloning efficiency is not high, it has recently been demonstrated that such cells grown in soft agar do retain markers characteristic of the original tumor cells (27). The possibility remains, however, that the cells which do grow are not a random selection of the tumor cells, but represent a more aggressive subset that may have a response to antitumor agents not characteristic of the whole tumor. Nevertheless, the soft agar culture system is one of the most important recent innovations in the area of screening systems for new antitumor agents.

The preceding general remarks outline the approach to the preclinical and initial clinical development of antitumor agents. A brief account of the development of three antitumor agents currently under active evaluation in the Grace Cancer Drug Center will be given to illustrate procedures and types of data being generated. The first of these, 2,4-diamino-5-adamantyl-6-methylpyrimidine, (DAMP), was synthesized and has undergone its entire preclinical development in the Grace Cancer Drug Center. The compound is presently awaiting an IND for initial clinical trial. The second compound, 3-deazauridine, was synthesized elsewhere, but has undergone its entire preclinical development, Phase I, and currently Phase II clinical trials, at the Roswell Park Memorial Institute. The third compound, a new platinum compound that was synthesized and underwent its initial preclinical evaluation in the United Kingdom, has been developed through large animal toxicology for clinical trial at the Roswell Park Memorial Institute. Preclinical studies on this compound are ongoing.

2,4-Diamino-5-Adamantyl-6-Methylpyrimidine (DAMP)

The structure of DAMP is shown in figure 1.2. The compound was synthesized by Zakrzewski and coworkers as one of a series of pyrimidines with lipophilic substituents in the 5-position designed to act as lipid-soluble inhibitors of dihydrofolate reductase (28), which might be free of some of the defects of methotrexate, such as lack of activity against many solid tumors, very poor penetration of the blood brain barrier necessitating its intrathecal administration to treat meningeal leukemia, and the rapid development of drug resistance. In the course of these studies, Zakrzewski and his coworkers showed that the structural requirements for inhibition of dihydrofolate reductase are the 2, 4-diaminopyrimidine moiety and the presence of a bulky, preferably lipophilic substituent at carbon 5 of the pyrimidine (18–32). The properties of DAMP are listed here.

1. Partition coefficient H_2O/n-heptane $= 17$ (as compared to 2,4-diamino-5,6-dimethyl pyrimidine $= 4,900$)
2. K_i for dihydrofolate reductase $= 6 \times 10^{-9}M$ (as compared to methotrexate $= 8 \times 10^{-10}M$)
3. ID_{50} for cultured TA3 cells $= 6 \times 10^{-9}M$ (as compared to MTX $= 8 \times 10^{-9}M$)
4. ID_{50} for cultured S180 cells resistant to methotrexate $4 \times 10^{-7}M$ (as compared to methotrexate $= 1.2 \times 10^{-5}M$)
5. Inhibition of W256, a tumor resistant to methotrexate 92% at 45 mg/kg $\times$ 5 I.P. (Zakrzewski et al. 28–33).

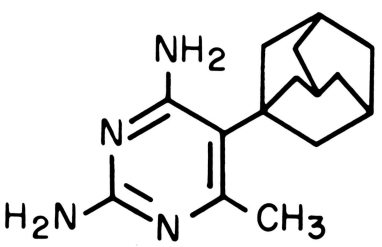

Fig. 1.2 Structure of 2,4-diamino-5-adamantyl-6-methylpyrimidine (DAMP)

It can be seen that the compound is lipid-soluble, has a K_i for dihydrofolate reductase comparable with that of methotrexate, an ID_{50} for cultured TA3 cells equivalent to that of methotrexate, and is effective against tumors which have both natural and acquired resistance to methotrexate.

The toxicity of DAMP has been studied in rodents and in large animals (33, 34). Its dose-limiting toxicity is gastrointestinal toxicity and myelosuppression, although it does not appear to show the marked specificity for megakaryocytes which characterized the related compound 2,4-diamino-5(3',4'-dichlorophenyl)-6-methylpyrimidine (DDMP) which caused difficulty in its extended clinical use (35). DAMP also shows some central nervous system (CNS) toxicity, which has been noted with other lipid-soluble antifols such as Bakers Antifol (triazinate), a substance which has been evaluated clinically by Bertino and coworkers (36).

Evaluation of the pharmacokinetics of DAMP in the rat, using the [^{14}C] labeled compound (37), showed a distribution into tissues, including brain, higher than that in plasma at all times up to 24 hr. Terminal phase half-life of total radioactivity in tissues is prolonged, although not as long as that in plasma. Studies on the metabolism of DAMP indicate that 20 min following I.V. administration, the bulk of the drug is in metabolite form in plasma, liver, and other tissues except brain. Even at two hours after I.V. administration, however, virtually all of the brain radioactivity is associated with unchanged DAMP (table 1.4).

Studies in the dog indicate that the short and long half-lives of unchanged DAMP are 31 and 411 min respectively (38). The volume of distribution is 125 l. At 24 hr, radioactivity in the urine is only 2.5% unaltered DAMP. Two metabolites have been found. One accounts for 12% of the urinary radioactivity, is relatively water-insoluble, and is extracted into organic solvents. The other, which is the major metabolite,

Table 1.4   Tissue Concentrations of Unchanged DAMP After [^{14}C] DAMP I.V. Administration in the Rat

Tissue	Concentration (plasma=1)		
	20 min	60 min	120 min
Liver	1.4	4.80	17.9
Brain	21.4	22.3	22.3
Kidney	18.0	25.7	23.1
Pancreas	8.4	11.0	7.6

SOURCE: Modified from Zakrzewski, Dave, and Rosen (33).

is water-soluble and remains in the aqueous layer after extraction with organic solvents.

The studies with DAMP thus far indicate that the pharmacokinetics of the drug are relatively consistent across species, giving us some confidence that these figures will not be unlike those which will be found clinically. The relatively short half-life and rapid metabolism of the drug is in contrast to some other diaminopyrimidine antifolates such as DDMP, and the fact that myelosuppression with DAMP is relatively easily reversible and does not show the characteristics of prolonged myelosuppression, particularly prolonged thrombocytopenia, which have characterized DDMP and made this drug difficult to use, are all features which give promise that this drug may have clinical potential, especially against methotrexate-resistant tumors. In addition, there is evidence that the drug crosses the blood brain barrier, making it a potential further treatment for brain tumors and meningeal leukemia.

3-Deazauridine (DAUR)

The structure of this compound is shown in figure 1.3. It is a structural analog of uridine, synthesized by Robins and Currie (39), in which the nitrogen in position 3 of the pyrimidine ring is replaced by carbon. It inhibits the growth of Ehrlich's ascites cells and L1210 cells in culture, producing 50% growth inhibition at a concentration of 6×10^{-6}M (40). It is also active against L1210 cells in vivo. In order to be active, the compound must be activated within the cell to the triphosphate DAUTP. In this form it acts as a competitive inhibitor of cytidine triphosphate (CTP) synthetase, the enzyme responsible for the conversion of uridine triphosphate (UTP) to CTP (41, 42), (figure 1.4).

Toxicological studies indicate that DAUR has primarily gastrointestinal toxicity in rodents, dogs, and monkeys, with hemorrhagic enterocolitis as the dose-limiting effect (34). Some degree of myelotoxicity is also seen (table 1.5). A feature of the toxicity of DAUR in rodents is an approximately twofold greater toxicity in female than in male mice, an effect which can be reversed by testosterone (table 1.6) (43).

The antitumor activity of DAUR was not markedly schedule dependent against a strain of leukemia L1210 sensitive to cytosine arabinoside (L1210/0). Marked schedule dependence was noted, however, against a strain resistant to cytosine arabinoside (L1210/ara-C) previously shown by Brockman to be much more sensitive to DAUR (44, 45, 46) (table 1.7). Studies of the uptake and activation of [14C] DAUR to [14C] DAUTP showed that DAUR was more extensively activated in the more sensitive cell line (L1210/ara-C) and that concentrations of the active metabolite were markedly higher up to two hours post treatment. The formation of

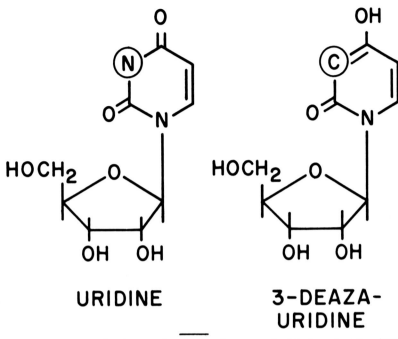

Fig. 1.3 Structure of 3-deazauridine (DAUR) compared with that of uridine (UR)

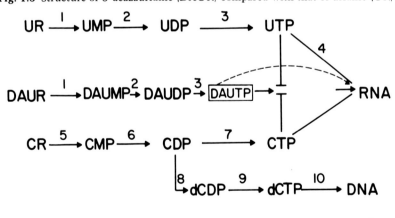

I. UR Kinase

2. UMP Kinase

3. UDP Kinase

4. RNA Polymerase

5. CR Kinase

6. CMP Kinase

7. CDP Kinase

8. Ribonucleotide Reductase

9. dCDP Kinase

I0. DNA Polymerase

Fig. 1.4 Metabolism of uridine (UR), cytidine (CR), and 3-deazauridine (DAUR) and the locus of action of DAUTP

Table 1.5   3-deazauridine (DAUR) Animal Toxicology

Degree of Toxicity	Toxic Effect
Major	Emesis
	Bloody diarrhea
	Loss of weight
Minor	Bone marrow depression
	Increase in liver enzymes and blood urea nitrogen
	Muscle weakness

SOURCE: Mihich et al. (34).

NOTE: Pathology: widespread necrosis of gastrointestinal tract. Lethal dose: 5,000 mg/m²/day × 5 in dog and monkey.

CTP from UTP was studied in the two cell lines. Formation of CTP from UPT in the L1210/ara-C cell line was half that in the L1210/0 cell line, perhaps indicating a lower level of the target enzyme for 3-deazauridine (46, 47, 48).

DAUR was more effective in female than in male mice (table 1.7). A study was therefore made of the pharmacokinetics of the drug, using [^{14}C] DAUR and chromatography to separate the parent drug from metabolites. The plasma decay curves for male and female mice are shown in figure 1.5. It can be seen that there is a marked and significant difference in levels at all the time points, related largely due to a slower absorption of the drug from the peritoneal cavity in male animals. This effect was partly reversed by testosterone (48).

Table 1.6   Effect of Testosterone on the Toxicity of 3-deazauridine (DAUR) in Female Mice

Testosterone (mg/mouse/day × 6)	Number Tested	30-Day Survivors
0.0	12	0
0.1	12	0
0.5	12	6
1.0	12	10
2.0	12	12

SOURCE: Bloch et al. (43).

NOTE: Female DBA$_2$/Ha mice received DAUR 250 mg/kg/day × 6 I.P. and testosterone subcutaneously.

Table 1.7 Response of L1210/0 and L1210/ara-C to 3-deazauridine (DAUR) in Female DBA2/CR Mice

	Percentage of Increase in Life Span*			Intracellular [^{14}C] DAUTP† (DPM/10^6 cells)			
	Schedule			Time (hr)			
Cell Line	A	B	C	0.5	1	2	4
L1210/0	30(0/10)‡	32(0/10)	32(0/10)	20.00	13.80	7.60	2.70
L1210/ Ara-C	62(0/10)	116(4/10)	160(7/10) [78(0/10)]§	68.60	46.00	22.40	12.80

SOURCE: Rustum et al. (45–47).
*Schedule A 43 mg/kg daily × 9
         B 96 mg/kg every 6 hr × 4
         C 48 mg/kg every 3 hr × 8
†After [^{14}C] DAUR I.V. at time zero.
‡Numbers in parentheses indicate long-term survivors of total treated.
§Male mice

In the Phase I study of DAUR, a starting dose of 400 mg/M^2/day for five days was used and the first dose escalation was 100%. Some biological effect was seen at 800 mg/M^2/day, so the escalation was reduced to 50%. 1,200 mg/M^2/day × 5 was the maximum tolerated dose in this study, although in one patient it was possible to increase it further. Eight of nine patients treated at this dose developed leucopenia, and four developed thrombocytopenia. The mean nadir of white blood count was 2,400/cu mm at day 15 (49).

Studies of the human pharmacokinetics of DAUR were carried out in patients receiving the drug as part of the Phase I study, using the [^{14}C] labeled drug. Separation of parent drug from metabolites was carried out using high-pressure liquid chromatography and paper chromatography. Recovery of radioactivity in the urine was nearly quantitative, and excretion was rapid (figure 1.6). Plasma decay of unchanged drug was biexponential, with a β phase t1/2 of 6.8 h. Plasma and urinary radioactivity were largely unchanged drug at the early time points, and 40–70% unchanged drug at later time points (50). This finding is in marked contrast to the data of Benvenuto and coworkers (51), who have studied the pharmacokinetics of unlabeled DAUR following continuous infusion of the drug and have found very extensive metabolism. The reason for this discrepancy is not yet clear.

The uptake and activation of [^{14}C] DAUR into leukemic blast cells of

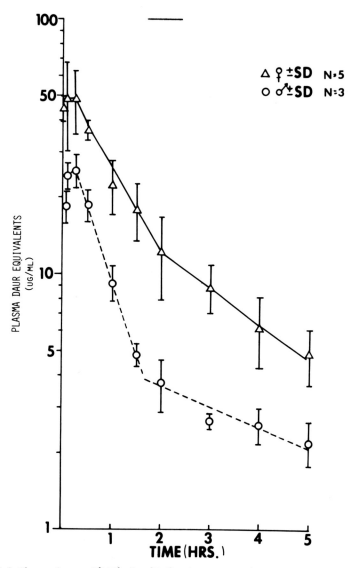

Fig. 1.5 Plasma decay of [^{14}C] after [^{14}C] 3-deazauridine (DAUR) I.P. in male and female DBA/2CR mice

patients with untreated acute myeloblastic leukemia were studied. A subset of patients (4 of 19) was found whose blast cell levels of DAUTP showed a mean value >4 standard deviations from the mean of the whole sample.

DAUR is now completing Phase II clinical trial in colon carcinoma at this institute.

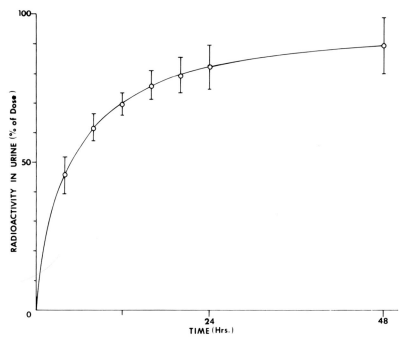

Fig. 1.6 Urinary recovery of [^{14}C] after 3-deazauridine (DAUR) I.V. in seven patients

Cis-dichloro-trans-dihydroxy-bis isopropylamine platinum [IV] (CHIP)

The third compound, which is currently undergoing intensive preclinical evaluation at the Grace Cancer Drug Center is a second-generation antitumor platinum complex. Cis-diamminedichloroplatinum-II (cisplatin) has shown marked clinical activity against a variety of tumors and has become a standard part of many therapeutic regimens for non-seminomatous testicular tumors. Its marked renal toxicity often limits its clinical usefulness, however, and requires the administration of intense hydration and often mannitol diuresis before adequate doses of the drug can be given. For this reason there is great interest in second-generation platinum compounds which, while retaining the therapeutic efficacy of cisplatin, are less nephrotoxic.

CHIP is a water-soluble platinum complex which, unlike cisplatin and most of the derivatives which have been examined to date, has platinum in the quadrivalent form. The compound has a high therapeutic ratio against the plasmacytoma PC6, which has been used by Connors to evaluate agents of this kind (52, 53). For this reason, we have studied both the toxicology and the pharmacokinetics of CHIP to determine whether it would 1) be less nephrotoxic and 2) show pharmacokinetics different from those of the parent drug. The structure of the compound is shown in figure 1.7. The pharmacokinetics of CHIP as compared to those of cisplatin as shown in table 1.8. It can be seen that CHIP has a shorter half-life than cisplatin, and although renal excretion is still incomplete, it is nevertheless greater at all time points than that of cisplatin (54, 55). Studies of the toxicity of CHIP and cisplatin in the rat show the hoped-for shift in the spectrum of toxicity. Cisplatin is primarily a nephrotoxic agent, whereas CHIP is primarily myelosuppressive (54, 55). For these reasons it is being developed for the clinic to determine whether it offers therapeutic benefits greater than those of the parent, cisplatin.

Conclusion

In this chapter we have attempted to summarize an approach to preclinical development and initial clinical testing of new antitumor agents, providing as an example the drug development program of the Grace Cancer Drug Center. This program, which integrates toxicological

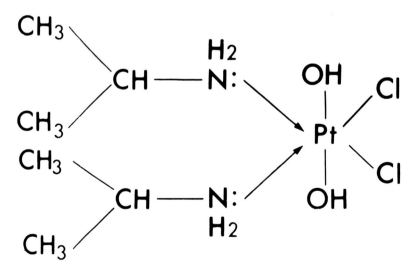

Fig. 1.7 Structure of cis-dichloro-trans-dihydroxy-bis isopropylamine platinum [IV] (CHIP)

Table 1.8   Pharmacokinetics of Pt. After CHIP and Cisplatin in the Rat

Drug	Plasma $t_{1/2}$		Urinary Excretion at 6 hr (Percentage of Dose)
	α (hr)	β (hr)	
CHIP	0.6	14	49.2
Cisplatin	—	69	35.6

SOURCE: Pfister et al. (54).

and antitumor efficacy data with pharmacological, pharmacokinetic, and biochemical data, aims at developing a full spectrum of information about the drug before it undergoes initial clinical trial. This body of information is expanded as the compound is used clinically. Data thus accumulated can then be used to develop dosages and schedules and to suggest specific tumor targets for which the drug might be valuable, drug combinations, and methods of modulating toxicity and antitumor efficacy, and to feed back to the drug development process to suggest the synthesis of newer analogs with greater efficacy and less toxicity. It is our belief that by this kind of integrated approach, in which a drug is tested in a clinical unit that is in close communication with those responsible for drug development, the potential of the large expenditure of manpower and resources invested in the development of new antitumor agents can be realized.

References

1. Schepartz, S. A. Screening. *Cancer Chemother. Rep.* Part 3, 2:3-8, 1971.

2. Wood, H. B., Jr. Selection of agents for the tumor screen. *Cancer Chemother. Rep.* Part 3, 2:9–22, 1971.

3. Chu, M. Y., and Fischer, G. A. A proposed mechanism of action of 1-β-D-arabinofuranosylcytosine as an inhibitor of the growth of leukemic cells. *Biochem. Pharmacol.* 11:423–430, 1962.

4. Cardeilhac, P. T., and Cohen, S. S. Some metabolic properties of nucleotides of 1-β-D-arabinofuranosylcytosine. *Cancer Res.* 24:1595–1603, 1964.

5. Arnold H., and Bourseaux, F. Synthese und Abbau cytostatisch wirksamer cyclischer N-Phosphain-idester des Bis-(β-chloräthyl)-amins. *Angew. Chem.* 70:539–544, 1958.

6. Foley, G. E.; Friedman, O. M.; and Drolet, B. P. Studies on the mechanism of action of cytoxan. Evidence of activation in vivo and in vitro. *Cancer Res.* 21:57–63, 1961.

7. Brock, N., and Hohorst, J. Über die aktivierung von cyklophosphamid in vivo und in vitro. *Arzneim. Forsch.* 12:1021–1031, 1963.

8. Rosenberg, B. et al. Platinum compounds: a new class of potent antitumour agent. *Nature* 222:385–386, 1969.

9. Creaven, P. J., and Mihich, E. The clinical toxicity of anticancer drugs and its prediction. *Semin. Oncol.* 4:147–163, 1977.

10. Creaven, P. J. Initial clinical trial of new anticancer drugs and extrapolation of animal data to man in preparation for clinical trials. Pp. 129–145 in *La chemioterapia dei tumori solidi*, vol. 2, ed. F. Pannuti. Bologna: Patron Press, 1979.

11. Mihich, E., and Grindey, G. B. Multiple basis of combination chemotherapy. *Cancer* 40:534–543, 1977.

12. Ensminger, W. D., and Frei, E. III. The prevention of methotrexate toxicity by thymidine infusions in humans. *Cancer Res.* 37:1857–1863, 1977.

13. Semon, J. H., and Grindey, G. B. Potentiation of the antitumor activity of methotrexate by concurrent infusion of thymidine. *Cancer Res.* 38:2905–2911, 1978.

14. Woodcock, T. M. et al. Phase I evaluation of thymidine plus flourouracil (TdR + FU) in patients with advanced cancer. *Proc. Am. Assoc. Cancer Res.* 19:351, 1978.

15. Mihich, E. Prediction of the potential toxicity of anticancer agents from studies in animals. Pp. 393–400 in *Methods in drug evaluation*, ed. P. Mantegazza and F. Piccinini. Amsterdam: North-Holland Publishing Co., 1966.

16. Creaven, P. J. Pharmacokinetic parameters: potential for and problems with their use as predictors of response to cancer chemotherapeutic agents. *Bull. Cancer* (Paris) 66:85–88, 1979.

17. This mouse was found by N. R. Grist *vide infra* reference 18.

18. Flanagan, S. P. "Nude," a new hairless gene with pleiotropic effects in the mouse. *Genet. Res.* 8:295, 1966.

19. Pantelouris, E. M. Absence of thymus in a mouse mutant. *Nature* 217:370–371, 1968.

20. Rygaard, J., and Povlsen, C. O. Heterotransplantation of a human malignant tumour to "nude" mice. *Acta Pathol. Microbiol. Scand.* 77:758–760, 1969.

21. Goldin, A. et al. Screening of anticancer drugs, historical development and current strategy of the National Cancer Institute Drug Development Program. Pp. 165–245 in *Methods in cancer research*, vol. XVI, *Cancer drug development part A*, ed. V. T. DeVita, Jr., and H. Busch. New York: Academic Press, Inc., 1979.

22. Park, C. H.; Bergsagel, D.; and McCulloch, E. Mouse myeloma tumor stem cells: a primary cell culture assay. *JNCI* 46:411–416, 1971.

23. Hamburger, A. W., and Salmon, S. E. Primary bioassay of human tumor stem cells. *Science* 197:461–463, 1977.

24. Hamburger, A., and Salmon, S. E. Primary bioassay of human myeloma stem cells. *J. Clin. Invest.* 60:846–854, 1977.

25. Salmon, S. E. et al. Quantitation of differential sensitivity of human-tumor stem cells to anticancer drugs. *N. Engl. J. Med.* 298:1321–1327, 1978.

26. Salmon, S. E. et al. Clinical correlations of drug sensitivity in tumor stem cell assay. P. 340 in *Proceedings: American Association for Cancer Research and American Society for Clinical Oncology Meetings*, vol. 20. Baltimore: Cancer Research, 1979.

27. Von Hoff, D. D., and Johnson, G. E. Secretion of tumor markers in the

human tumor stem cell system. P. 51 in *Proceedings: American Association for Cancer Research and American Society for Clinical Oncology Meetings*, vol. 20. Baltimore: Cancer Research, 1979.

28. Jonak, J. P.; Zakrzewski, S. F.; and Mead, L. H. Synthesis and biological activity of some 5-(1-adamantyl) pyrimidines. *J. Med. Chem.* 14:408, 1971.

29. Jonak, J. P.; Zakrzewski, S. F.; and Mead, L. H. Synthesis and biological activity of some 5-substituted 2,4-diamino-6-alkylpyrimidines. *J. Med. Chem.* 15:662, 1972.

30. Ho, Y. K.; Hakala, M. T.; and Zakrzewski, S. F. 5-(1-adamantyl) pyrimidines as inhibitors of folate metabolism. *Cancer Res.* 32:1023–1028, 1972.

31. Jonak, J. P. et al. Effect of the substituent at C-6 on the biological activity of 2,4-diamino-5-(1-adamantyl) pyrimidines. *J. Med. Chem.* 16:724-725, 1973.

32. Ho, Y. K.; Zakrzewski, S. F.; and Mead, L. H. Hydrophobic interactions between the 5-alkyl group of 2,4-diamino-6-methylpyrimidines and dihydrofolate reductase. *Biochemistry* 12:1003–1005, 1973.

33. Zakrzewski, S. F.; Dave, C.; and Rosen, F. Comparison of the antitumor activity and toxicity of 2,4-diamino-5-(1-adamantyl)-6-methylpyrimidine and 2,4-diamino-5-(1-adamantyl)-6-ethylpyrimidine. *JNCI* 60:1029–1033, 1978.

34. Mihich, E. M. et al., unpublished data.

35. Murphy, M. L. et al. Clinical effects of the dichloro and monochlorophenyl analogs of diamino pyrimidine: antagonists of folic acid. *J. Clin. Invest.* 33:1388–1396, 1954.

36. Skeel, R. T. et al. Clinical and pharmacological evaluation of triazinate in humans. *Cancer Res.* 36:48–54, 1976.

37. Zakrzewski, S. F. et al. Studies with a new antifolate 2,4-diamino-5-adamantyl-6-methylpyrimidine (DAMP): tissue distribution and disposition of 2,4-diamino-5-adamantyl-6-methylpyrimidine and its metabolite. *J. Pharmacol. Exp. Ther.* 205:19–26, 1978.

38. Zakrzewski, S. F., and Creaven, P. J. Pharmacokinetics of 2,4-diamino-5-adamantyl-6-methyl pyrimidine (DAMP) in Dogs. P. 225 in *Proceedings: American Association for Cancer Research and American Society for Clinical Oncology Meetings*, vol. 20. Baltimore: Cancer Research, 1979.

39. Robins, M. J., and Currie, B. L. The synthesis of 3-deazauridine [4-hydroxy-1-(β-D-ribopentofuranosyl)-2-pyridine]. *Chem. Comm.* 2:1547–1548, 1968.

40. Bloch, A. et al. Preparation and biological activity of various 3-deazapyrimidines and related nucleosides. *J. Med. Chem.* 16:294–297, 1973.

41. Wang, M. C., and Bloch, A. Studies on the mode of action 3-deazapyridimines—I metabolism of 3-deazauridine and 3-deazacytidine in microbial and tumor cells. *Biochem. Pharmacol.* 21:1063–1073, 1972.

42. McPartland, R. P. et al. Cytidine 5'triphosphate synthetase as a target for inhibition by the antitumor agent 3-deazauridine. *Cancer Res.* 34:3107–3111, 1974.

43. Bloch, A. et al. Prevention by testosterone of the intestinal toxicity caused by the antitumor agent 3-deazauridine. *Cancer Res.* 34:1299–1303, 1974.

44. Brockman, R. W. et al. The mechanism of action of 3-deazauridine in

tumor cells sensitive and resistant to arabinosyl-cytosine. *Ann. NY Acad. Sci.* 225:501–521, 1975.

45. Rustum, Y. M., and Creaven, P. J. Studies on the antitumor activity of 3-deazauridine (DAUR) against mouse leukemia L1210 sensitive to (L1210/0) and resistant to (L1210/ara-C) cytosine arabinoside. *Fed. Proc.* 36:355, 1977.

46. Rustum, Y. M.; Creaven, P. J.; and Slocum, H. K. Biochemical and pharmacological studies of 3-deazauridine with L1210 sensitive and resistant to cytosine arabinoside. Pp. 1118–1120 in *Current chemotherapy. Proceedings of the 10th International Congress of Chemotherapy*, vol. 2, ed. W. Siegenthaler and R. Luthy. Washington, D.C.: American Society for Microbiology, 1978.

47. Rustum, Y. M., and Creaven, P. J. Studies on the antitumor activity of 3-deazauridine (DAUR) against mouse leukemia L1210 sensitive to (L1210/0) and resistant to (L1210/ara-C) cytosine arabinoside. *Fed. Proc.* 36:355, 1977.

48. Slocum, H. K.; Rustum, Y. M.; and Creaven, P. J. Sex differences in pharmacokinetics and antitumor activity of 3-deazauridine (DAUR) in mice. P. 85 in *Proceedings: American Association for Cancer Research and American Society for Clinical Oncology Meetings*, vol. 19. Baltimore: Cancer Research, 1978.

49. Creaven, P. J. Initial clinical trial of 3-deazauridine (DAUR). Abs. 12th Intl. Cancer Congress, Buenos Aires, Argentina, 1:305, 1978.

50. Creaven, P. J. et al. The clinical pharmacokinetics of 3-deazauridine, a new antineoplastic agent. Pp. 1208–1210 in *Current chemotherapy. Proceedings of the 10th International Congress of Chemotherapy*, vol. 2, ed. W. Siegenthaler and R. Luthy. Washington, D.C.: American Society for Microbiology, 1978.

51. Benvenuto, J. A. et al. Pharmacokinetics and disposition of 3-deazauridine in humans. *Cancer Res.* 39:349–352, 1979.

52. Braddock, P. D. et al. Structure and activity relationships of platinum complexes with anti-tumour activity. *Chem. Biol. Interact.* 11:145–161, 1975.

53. Wilkinson, R. et al. Selection of potential second generation platinum compounds. *Biochimie* 60:851–857, 1978.

54. Pfister, M. et al. Dichlorodihydroxybisisopropylamine platinum IV a new antitumor platinum complex. Pharmacokinetics in the rat: relation to renal toxicity. *Biochimie* 60:1057–1058, 1978.

55. Mihich, E. et al. Preclinical studies of dihydroxy-cis-dichloro-bis-iso-propylamine platinum IV (CHIP). Proceedings: American Association for Cancer Research and American Society for Clinical Oncology Meetings, vol. 20:426, 1979.

Chapter 2

Biochemical and Pharmacological Determinants of Drug Action

Youcef M. Rustum, Ph.D.
Lynn Danhauser
Harvey Preisler, M.D.
Arnold Mittelman, M.D.
and Elihu Ledezma, M.D.

Parameters of Drug Action

In the last several years, numerous laboratories have been involved in evaluating parameters that may aid in predicting the response of tumor cells to antimetabolites, specifically cytosine arabinoside (ara-C) and 5-fluorouracil (FU). In the case of ara-C, these parameters include plasma half-life of the intact drug, phosphorylation of the nucleoside to the presumed active component, namely the triphosphate of ara-C (ara-CTP), incorporation of the drug into nucleic acids, determination of the intracellular concentration of the natural metabolite, and monitoring of the deoxycytidine (CdR) kinase to CdR deaminase ratio. The results of these studies have shown that evaluation of a single parameter is insufficient to predict the sensitivity of tumor cells to the drug.

An additional parameter that may aid in determining the activity of ara-C and other antimetabolites is the intracellular nucleotide (ribo- and deoxyribonucleotide) pools. The rationale for evaluating the nucleotides as predictors of response is that at different stages of antimetabolite activation the antimetabolite pools equilibrate with metabolic pools and, in turn, affect those pools through inhibition exerted at one or more specific enzymatic reactions along a particular pathway (1, 2). The interplay between the size of the metabolite pools and antimetabolite action is complicated by the fact that certain critical pools (ribo- and deoxyribonucleotides) act as regulators of metabolic pathways. Thus, the nucleotide pool profile may be an inherent characteristic of a particular tumor, cell type, or particular stage of tumor pathology (2, 3).

Another parameter that should be considered in predicting tumor cell sensitivity is the plasma level of nucleosides and bases, specifically those metabolites that are the natural counterparts of the antimetabolites under investigation (e.g., CdR versus ara-C). The rationale for evaluating plasma levels of nucleosides and bases is that 1) these metabolites most likely share a common mechanism with corresponding antimetabolites for uptake into cells, and 2) they may alter specific intracellular metabolic pools which compete with the active form of the antimetabolite at its critical site of action or which provide end products of the inhibited reaction. Indeed, increased serum levels of these metabolites (caused by cell destruction, diet modification, and so forth) will undoubtedly affect the cellular uptake of the corresponding antimetabolite and may render target cells insensitive to that particular agent. For instance, based upon the original observations of Hakala (4, 5) and numerous subsequent studies in culture with a variety of cell lines, it is now apparent that thymidine and a purine (e.g., hypoxanthine) may contribute to a different extent to the reversal of methotrexate-induced cytotoxicity, depending on the cell type studied (4). Thus the opportunity might be afforded in vivo to differentially alter methotrexate toxicity by providing the salvage precursor of a pool that may be limiting in a normal target tissue but not in the tumor. The recent reports of increased therapeutic effectiveness of high doses of methotrexate in combination with thymidine in human beings (6) and in mice (7, 8) attest to this possibility. These studies provide evidence that normal metabolites may indeed play a role in determining the selectivity of action of antimetabolites. Further studies are needed to document the levels of relevant metabolites in the plasma of patients with acute myelocytic leukemia (AML) prior to or during treatment and to evaluate the role of these salvage metabolites in clinical anticancer therapy.

In view of the preceding considerations, it can be understood why examination of a single or even a few parameters of drug action may not provide enough predictive information on tumor sensitivity. Selected parameters such as drug uptake, however, may predict for intrinsic tumor insensitivity. A multiplicity of factors must be evaluated in order to assess tumor sensitivity in individual patients and, in most cases, a selection of the most critical parameters cannot be made at the outset. Indeed, target cell determinants may vary among tumor masses at different sites in the same patient. Presumably, increased knowledge of the action of drugs in sensitive and resistant tumors may allow for more rational use of drugs in the treatment of human malignancy.

It is apparent that the lethal action of drugs in target cells depends on numerous interactions among many factors operating in the whole organism as well as in the target cell itself. In this chapter, we will describe factors affecting cellular response to FU and ara-C and discuss how these factors may be modified by normal metabolites.

Metabolism of Fluorinated-(F)-Pyrimidines by Tumor Cells

The determinants of FU action for predicting cellular response may depend on the balance of two major pathways: the anabolic and the catabolic pathways. The anabolic pathway leads to the formation of 5-fluoro-2'-deoxyuridine-5'-monophosphate (FdUMP) and to the eventual incorporation of the drug into RNA, while the catabolic pathway leads to a shorter half-life and a lower plasma level of the intact drug and, consequently, to lower anabolic activities. Kessel and Hall (9) demonstrated that, in a number of rodent tumors, anabolism of FU to the nucleotide level correlated with enhanced response to the drug. Wolberg (10) and Klubes (11) have shown that inhibition of deoxyuridine, thymidine, and formate incorporation into DNA was not predictive for response to FU.

In [comparing] L1210 cells sensitive (L1210/0) and resistant to FUR (L1210/FUR), both the pools of FdUMP and incorporation into RNA were reported higher in the sensitive than in the resistant tumor cells (12). On the other hand, in comparisons of these parameters in L1210/0 and in L1210/FUR when FU was used, the pools of FdUMP and the incorporation of the drug into RNA were, by themselves, insufficient to explain the difference in the response of the two cell lines. The resistant tumor was totally unresponsive to FUR, while the sensitive tumor yielded a 50% increase in the life spans of mice treated with FU and a greater than 200% increase in the life spans of mice treated with FUR. Klubes and his coworkers (13) have shown that although the initial level of FdUMP in the FU-resistant Walker 256 tumor was higher than that found in sensitive L1210 cells, at 48 hr following drug administration the level of FdUMP in the resistant tumor was no longer detectable. In responsive solid L1210 tumor cell, sensitivity correlated with longer retention of FdUMP in tumor cells.

In vitro studies have been carried out to determine the ability of tumor cells obtained from the peripheral blood of patients with AML to take up and incorporate F-pyrimidines into RNA. The results obtained, summarized in figure 2.1, show wide quantitative variability among patients in the way F-pyrimidines are handled by leukemic cells. In general, the uptake into the acid-soluble fraction was in the order of FUR > FUdR >

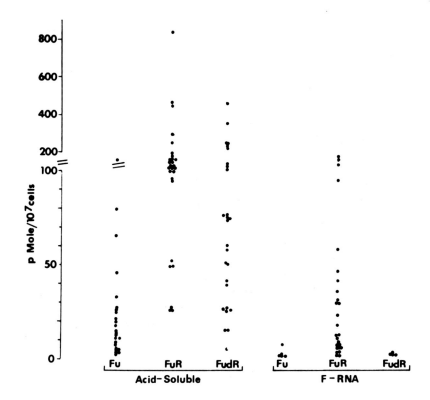

Fig. 2.1 Uptake into the acid-soluble fraction and incorporation into RNA of fluorinated-(F)-pyrimidine by leukemic cells obtained from peripheral blood of patients with acute myelocytic leukemia (AML). Cells (5.0–10.0 × 10⁶ cells) were incubated with FU-2-[¹⁴C] (5 μCi), FUR-2-[¹⁴C] (2.5 μCi) or FUdR-2-[¹⁴C] (5 μCi) for 30 min at 37°C in the presence of Roswell Park Memorial Institute (RPMI) 1640 containing 10% fetal calf serum. Total radioactivity found in the acid-soluble fraction and the amount of drug incorporated into RNA were quantitated.

FU. The incorporation into RNA, however, was greatest when FUR was used. The incorporation of FU and fluorodeoxyuridine (FUdR) into RNA was greater than 1 pmole/m² in only 4 of 24 and 4 of 26 patients respectively. Preliminary results indicated that the level of FdUMP in the acid-soluble fraction was the highest when FUdR was used. In fact, in some cases over 90% of the acid-soluble counts derived from FUdR were in the form of FdUMP.

These in vitro data suggest that the rate of FUdR conversion to FU and its subsequent incorporation into RNA is relatively slow in target AML cells. Since the systemic degradation and elimination of FUdR are rapid, and since leukemic cells have the ability to take up and activate FUdR to FdUMP, correlation between the rate of conversion of FUdR to FdUMP with clinical response to FUdR should be evaluated. In contrast, the consequences of F-pyrimidine incorporation into RNA by AML cells may be evaluated using FUR as the agent of choice instead of FUdR.

The uptake of FUdR into acid-soluble pools and incorporation of the drug into RNA by "normal" liver and liver metastases from colon carcinoma were investigated. These patients all had massive (> 70%) liver metastases from a colonic primary, but had no other known site of neoplastic involvement. The FUdR (25 mg containing 500 μCi [³H] FUdR) was injected through the hepatic artery, proven to be the main source of blood supply to metastatic tumoral cells (14, 15, 16), and samples of both normal liver parenchyma and tumor were taken at 30–60 min. Rapid freezing was applied to all samples. Perchloric acid-soluble and -insoluble fractions (RNA) were then isolated, and their radioactive content determined. Table 2.1 summarizes the data obtained in specimens from seven patients. The data indicated that in two of six patients, the amount of FUdR incorporated into the RNA of normal liver tissues (presumably by conversion of FUdR to FU with subsequent phosphorylation) was less than that incorporated by tumor cells. The amount of radioactivity found in the acid-soluble fraction varied considerably. In three of the seven patients, the acid-soluble pool of label derived from FUdR was higher in normal tissues, except for the liver and tumor tissues in patient 7. These preliminary results indicated a wide variation in the degree of uptake and activation of FUdR. Studies are currently under way to identify the various FUdR metabolites found in the acid-soluble fraction and to determine whether or not the same degree of heterogeneity exists [as is found in normal vs.] solid tumor tissues. Some degree of selectivity for FUdR might exist in patients whose tumor cells exhibit greater uptake of this agent than do their adjacent normal tissues.

In order to quantitate the various factors involved in the effectiveness of FU, studies were initiated using L1210 cells sensitive and resistant to each of the F-pyrimidines, namely FU, FUR, and FUdR. The data summarized in table 2.2 indicate that 1) the total uptake of F-pyrimidines in both cell lines was in the order of FUR > FUdR > FU, 2) the uptake of F-pyrimidines by resistant tumor cells was several times less than that of the sensitive cell line, and 3) the pool of FdUMP in both cell lines was largest when derived from FUR, but was significantly lower in the resistant cell lines. Incorporation into RNA was highest in both lines when FUR was used, while the differences between the sensitive and resistant cell lines when FU or FUdR were employed were much less significant. Although

Table 2.1   Uptake and incorporation of fluorodeoxyuridine (FUdR) into RNA by normal and tumor tissues obtained from patients with colon carcinoma

| Patient | Sample | pmole/gm Tissue | |
		Acid-soluble Fractions	RNA
1	tumor	354	95
	normal	2,565	249
2	tumor	390	ND*
	normal	1,466	ND
3	tumor	181	259
	normal	138	506
4	tumor	437	243
	normal	738	165
5	tumor	6,967	551
	normal	1,089	214
6	tumor	12,255	4,421
	normal	3,943	2,157
7	tumor	128	391

NOTE: Thirty to 60 min prior to surgery, FUdR (25 mg containing 500 μCi[^{3}H] FUdR) were injected via the hepatic vein. Tumor and adjacent normal liver tissue were removed and frozen rapidly. Perchloric acid-soluble and-insoluble fractions (RNA) were then isolated and their content of radioactivity determined.

*ND = not determined.

L1210/FU cells in vivo are totally resistant to F-pyrimidines, the sensitivity of L1210/0 in vivo was in the order of FUR > FU > FUdR. If FdUMP concentration is the only critical factor determining the sensitivity of L1210 cells to F-pyrimidines, then mice bearing L1210/0 should be more sensitive to FUdR than to FU. The pools of FdUMP derived from FUdR and FU were 131 and 5.1 pmoles/10^7 cells respectively. Furthermore, although the pools of FdUMP derived from FUdR in L1210/FU (22.0 pmoles/10^7 cells) were significantly higher than those derived from FU in L1210/0, L1210/FU cells were totally resistant to FUdR.

Regarding the incorporation of F-pyrimidines into RNA, the data presented in table 2.2 indicate that the level of FUR incorporation into RNA by L1210/FU was greater than the incorporation of FU into RNA by L1210/0. These data indicate that the sensitivity of L1210 cells to F-pyrimidines depends on factors other than the initial pool of FdUMP and incorporation into RNA. Hence evaluation of other factors such as FdUMP retention, the level of thymidylate synthetase, the level of the competing substrate, dUMP, and pharmacokinetic parameters collectively may be more critical in predicting the sensitivity of tumor cells to F-pyrimidines.

The value of pharmacokinetics as the sole determinant of the selectivity of antitumor action is questionable. It is conceivable, however, that pharmacokinetics may contribute to FU selectivity of action in conjunction with other determinants of drug action. Indeed, depending on cell metabolism and the pharmacology at the target cell level, a given concentration of a drug attained for a certain period of time may be sufficient to affect one cell type and not another. Attempts to modify the pharmacokinetic and target cell determinants of the action of FU and other agents will be discussed in more detail later in this chapter.

Target Determinants of ara-C Action in Leukemia

At the present time, the choice of drugs to be given to an individual patient with a specific type of tumor is still largely empirical. Decisions are made on the basis of information about responses obtained in other patients with that type of tumor, in spite of the fact that individual responses vary widely among those patients. This approach is, neverthe-

Table 2.2 In vivo uptake and activation of F-pyrimidines by leukemia L1210 cells sensitive (L1210/0) and resistant (L1210/FU) to FU

| Precursors | $pmole/10^7$ Cells | | | | $pmole/\mu g$ RNA | |
| | Acid-soluble | | FdUMP | | F-RNA | |
	L1210/0	L1210/FU	L1210/0	L1210/FU	L1210/0	L1210/FU
FU	31.0	17.7	5.1	3.2	0.5	0.4
FUR	9071.0	1215.0	575.0	49.0	37.5	6.6
FUdR	592.0	151.0	131.0	22.0	0.5	0.3

NOTE: DBA/2J mice bearing four-day-old tumors were treated with therapeutic doses of 100 mg/kg of FU, 200 mg/kg FUdR, or 10 mg/kg FUR, each containing a tracer dose of labeled drug (10 μCi/mouse). One hour following treatment, cells were removed and extracted and the intracellular drug metabolites were quantitated by high-pressure liquid chromatography.

less, the best available. Only when enough information on the mode of action of drugs in human beings is acquired to permit the formulation of reasonable assumptions about the probable pharmacological and biochemical determinants of selectivity in the individual patient will it be possible to "tailor" the choice of drugs to the characteristics of the specific tumor.

In recent years, highly potent drugs have become available for the treatment of AML, namely ara-C in combination with the anthracyclines adriamycin and daunorubicin. This has resulted in an overall complete remission rate of 60–70%, with a remission rate of 80% in patients under 60 years of age (17–19). The therapy is administered to virtually all AML patients and all become severely pancytopenic with associated infections. While the therapy is successful with respect to remission induction for patients under 60 years of age, about 20% of these patients might have been better off with some other form of therapy. At the present time, it cannot be clinically ascertained which patients should not receive the current induction therapy of ara-C plus adriamycin. Clinical parameters by themselves are inadequate bases for this determination. There are subgroups of patients, however, who cannot be identified on an individual basis and who respond less adequately to the present method of therapy. These patients should clearly not be treated in an identical fashion to those patients with curative potential on the present therapeutic regimen. Unfortunately, our inability to identify such patients prevents us from giving alternative forms of therapy. The existence of variable responses to chemotherapy among patient subpopulations presents a problem in the therapy of virtually all neoplastic diseases.

Acute leukemia has a unique feature which makes it an ideal neoplastic disease in which to test the proposition that it is possible to distinguish individuals who are likely to respond to a particular chemotherapeutic regimen from those who are not. This feature is that we can repeatedly obtain large numbers of viable leukemic cells at little or no risk to the health of the patient. The accessibility of leukemic cells has permitted the development of methodologies for the simultaneous evaluation of multiple critical parameters of drug action in individual patients prior to and during therapy.

Several potential target cell determinants of ara-C action may be identified based upon current knowledge of its mechanism of action. Since ara-C requires activation to ara-CTP in target cells in order to exert its activity on DNA polymerase, the size of the pools of ara-CTP in AML cells should provide a good indication of ara-C entry into the cells and of its metabolic activation. Because the action of a drug usually depends not only on the concentration of active drug that reaches the proximal site of action but also on the length of time during which effective drug concentrations are retained at this site, the retention of ara-CTP in AML cells may be a determinant of drug action. The formation of ara-CTP may be affected by the extent of ara-C deamination within the target cells and by the metabolic regulation of target cells as reflected by the profile of ribo- and deoxyribonucleotide pools and the preferential utilization of de novo versus salvage pathways of nucleotide synthesis. In addition, the effectiveness of the ara-CTP formed is likely to be affected by the rate of DNA synthesis and related requirements for DNA polymerase activity in the target cells. The relevance of some of these determinants to the therapeutic effects of ara-C in patients with AML has been verified (20–22).

Intracellular Pools and Retention of the Active Form of Antimetabolites

Correlation between the intracellular pools, retention of ara-CTP and therapeutic response.

Studies have now been carried out to determine the intracellular concentration and the retention time of ara-CTP in L1210, P288, and Taper hepatoma cells in vivo (22). These factors appear to be the most important parameters in predicting the response of the three tumor cell lines in vivo. In all three tumors, the drug was metabolized to the triphosphate level and the amount of the 5′monophosphate of 1-β-D-arabinofuranosyluracil (ara-UMP) formed was similar, but relatively small. The amount of ara-CTP formed and retained in the cells, however, was largest in L1210 and smallest in Taper hepatoma: the intracellular pools of ara-CTP in L1210 cells were 10- and 20-fold greater than those found in P288 and Taper hepatoma cells, respectively. The highest ara-CTP level in L1210 and P288 or Taper hepatoma cells was observed at 15 and 60 min, respectively after application of the labeled nucleoside. In the Taper hepatoma, the 5′monophosphate of ara-C (ara-CMP) pools were, at all time points, significantly larger than those found in L1210 or P288 cells. Similar results were obtained when these cells were incubated with [5-^{3}H] ara-C in vitro. Furthermore, the level of ara-CTP in L1210 cells was compared to that attained in host small intestine and spleen. In L1210, the half-life of ara-CTP was about six hours, but less than 2 hours in the small intestine or spleen. Four hours after I.V. administration of ara-C, ara-CTP levels were 24.6, 3.2, and 1.2 nmoles/gm in L1210, small intestine, and spleen, respectively.

Based upon these data, the schedule of administration of ara-C to mice bearing L1210, P288, and Taper hepatoma was examined. The best results were obtained by injecting 6 doses of 20 mg/kg every four hours. Using this schedule, 8 of 15 mice bearing L1210 survived longer than 60 days, while only 68 and 18% increases in survival time were obtained for P288 and Taper hepatoma, respectively. Treatment with 12 doses of 10 mg/kg every two hours produced marked toxicity and no significant antitumor activity in all cell lines. These data suggest that the differences in sensitivity of these tumors seem related to the differential net tissue levels of ara-CTP and its duration of retention at the target site (22).

The aforementioned studies were extended to investigate ara-C metabolism in AML cells obtained from 28 individual patients to determine whether the parameters identified for the prediction of response in the three mouse tumors could be equally predictable in the human situation (21, 22). The results of this study indicated that first, whenever ara-C was taken up by AML cells in vitro it was phosphorylated to the triphosphate level, namely ara-CTP, and became incorporated into macromolecules. In a few cases, however, there was no significant uptake and activation of ara-C when cells were incubated in vitro with 1–10 mM ara-C for up to two hours. Second, there were quantitative differences between patients in the amount of ara-CTP initially formed that was retained intracellularly at four hours. Consistent with earlier observations in mice, the pools of ara-UMP did not fluctuate significantly in cells obtained from patients with AML. On the basis of these differences, the patients could be placed into two subgroups: those 13 patients whose leukemic cell retention was > 36%, and the remaining 15 patients whose leukemic cells retained < 19% of the ara-CTP. Of the 13 patients in the high-retention group, 11 attained complete remission with 8 requiring a single course of therapy. Seven of the 11 patients remained in complete remission from 55 to > 129 weeks. Nine of the 15 patients whose ara-CTP retention was < 19% attained complete remission with 3 requiring two courses of therapy. Eight of these patients relapsed between 11 and 92 weeks, with a single patient remaining in remission at > 58 weeks. The median remission duration for the low-retention group was 28 weeks, while that of the high-retention group exceeded 63 weeks.

These data indicate that although these patients were clinically diagnosed as having AML and were treated in an identical manner, their cells metabolized ara-C differently. The data demonstrate a significant correlation between ara-CTP formation and retention in vitro by AML cells and the duration of remission in patients receiving ara-C as part of their remission induction and maintenance therapy.

Plasma Deamination of ara-C to 1-β-D-arabinofuranosyluracil (ara-U)

Another parameter used for the in vitro characterization of patients with AML was the ability of the patient's own plasma to deaminate ara-C to ara-U. To date, we have analyzed plasma obtained from 8 normal individuals and 20 patients with AML and the results are summarized in table 2.3.

To obtain the data presented in table 2.3, plasma from each individual (prior to therapy) was incubated with [5-^{3}H] ara-C, and at 5, 20, and 60 min thereafter aliquots were removed, deproteinized, and analyzed by high-pressure liquid chromatography for the extent of ara-U formation. In normal individuals, after 60 min of incubation the amount of ara-C ranged from 72–94%, with a mean value of 88%. In 75% of the AML patients analyzed, ara-C was the dominant component found. After 60 min of incubation, the values ranged from 88–94% with a mean value of 89%. In 25% of the patients' plasma, however, there was a rapid deamination of ara-C to ara-U, with 71% of the label appearing in the form of ara-U. The extent of ara-C conversion to ara-U was analyzed in "fresh" plasma and compared with that of plasma kept for several days at −72°C. The results indicated that there was no significant difference between the two methods in the amount of ara-U formed.

These results indicate that while the majority of patients with AML do not significantly catabolize ara-C in their plasma, a small number of patients seem to have high CdR deaminase levels and, consequently, their tumor cells are probably exposed to ineffective levels of ara-C. Hence, to develop an effective in vitro predictive assay for ara-C sensitivity based on the metabolism of AML cells, the procedure must be designed to take into consideration the variation in plasma levels of ara-C observed in different patients.

Modulation of the Toxicity and Antitumor Activity of FU by Normal Metabolites

Studies were carried out to evaluate the therapeutic efficacy of FU when administered in combination with normal purine and pyrimidine metabolites. These studies were carried out in normal (untumored) Balb/C and C57BL/6J mice and in caesarean-delivered Fischer (CDF) rats. Normal metabolites alone or in combination with FU were infused I.V. for 72 hr (23, 24). The results indicated that infusion of up to 10 gm/kg of thymidine, inosine, uridine, deoxyinosine, or deoxyribose was not toxic to the host. The lethal doses of FU in rats and mice are listed in table 2.4 (25).

Table 2.3   In vitro deamination of ara-C to ara-U by human plasma obtained from normal individuals and from patients with acute myelocytic leukemia (AML)

Cases	Disease State	Percentage of ara-C		Percentage of ara-U	
		Range	Mean	Range	Mean
8	Normal	72–94	88	6–28	12
15	AML, low apparent deaminase	88–94	89	6–12	11
5	AML, high apparent deaminase	27–31	29	69–73	71

NOTE: Five ml of plasma were incubated at 37°C with labeled ara-C and, at 5, 20, and 60 min therafter, serum was prepared for ara-C and ara-U analysis. Only the data for the 60-min incubation are shown in the table.

Infusion of FU at the lethal dose for 50% of the animals (LD$_{50}$) alone caused gastrointestinal toxicity, necrosis of the liver and spleen, hemorrhage of the adrenals and lymph nodes, and degenerative changes of the kidney. Infusion of FU at the LD$_0$ showed no toxicity other than weight loss. The LD$_0$ of FU became LD$_{75}$ if it was infused together with thymidine, inosine, uridine, deoxyinosine, or deoxyribose at doses of 5 gm/kg/72 hr. These combinations resulted in similar pathology to that observed using the LD$_{50}$ or LD$_{100}$ of FU alone. These studies also show that, in general, infusion of 5 gm/kg/72 hr of metabolite together with FU potentiates the toxicity of FU in this order in both rats and mice, although to varying degrees: the toxicity of uridine is greater than or equal to that of thymidine, which is in turn greater than that of inosine. Initial results seem to indicate that a correlation exists between the plasma levels of

Table 2.4   Lethal doses of fluorouracil (FU) in rats and mice obtained by 72-hr continuous I.V. infusion.

Strain	Lethal Doses (mg/kg/72 hr)		
	0%	50%	100%
CDF rats	150	350	450
Balb/C mice	125	225	400
C57BL/65 mice	175	350	500

normal metabolites in different hosts and the amount of thymidine required to potentiate the toxicity of FU. For example, in C57BL/6J mice in which the normal metabolite level in plasma was low, more thymidine was required to induce toxicity comparable to that observed in Balb/C mice or in CDF rats using a lower thymidine concentration. These data suggest that the plasma level of normal purine and pyrimidine metabolites might influence the amount of thymidine or FU required to induce comparable toxicity in different individuals. For this reason, metabolite levels should be quantitated before and during therapy with anti-metabolite-metabolite combinations.

The antitumor activity of FU alone or in combination with 5 gm/kg of thymidine or uridine was evaluated against subcutaneous mouse and rat colon tumors by comparing the effects of the maximally tolerated dose (MTD) of FU when administered by I.V. bolus or by 72-hr infusion (26). In tumor-bearing rats, infusion (150 mg/kg) or I.V. bolus administration (200 mg/kg) of FU inhibited tumor growth by 94–100% in controls, with no significant difference in increase in life span. Infusion of FU (100 mg/kg) in combination with thymidine resulted in complete tumor regression in all animals (12 of 12) with a 45% increase in life span (7 of 12). In addition, 5 of the 12 rats were tumor-free 150 days posttreatment (controls died after 60–80 days). Thymidine administered by infusion or I.V. bolus did not yield significant increases in life span. Preliminary studies in rats indicated that concurrent infusion of uridine with FU (35 mg/kg) produced anti-tumor activity similar to that of the thymidine combination. In mice bearing colon tumor no. 26, there was little difference in tumor reduction (60–70%) between FU infusion, bolus FU, or FU combined with thymidine. Initial results, however, suggested that coinfusion of thymidine and FU (100 mg/kg) produced a 43% increase in life span, while bolus administration of FU alone (90 mg/kg) produced only a 14% increase in life span.

These results can be summarized as follows:

1. Normal metabolites dramatically potentiated the toxicity of FU in rodents.
2. The MTD of FU alone or in combination with thymidine in mice bearing colon tumor no. 26 produced no significant increase in life span and no long-term survivors.
3. Infusion of thymidine with FU at the MTD resulted in more tumor-free survivors than infusion or I.V. bolus of FU alone in rats bearing colon carcinoma.
4. The combinations of thymidine or uridine with FU at the MTD were equally effective against rat colon tumor.

The effects of nucleosides and bases on the plasma interconversion of

FU, FUR, and FUdR were evaluated in DBA/2J mice following an I.V. bolus injection of metabolites (27). The data indicate that 1) nucleosides in the plasma can serve as ribose or deoxyribose donors for the conversion of FU to FUR and FUdR respectively; 2) bases minimize the metabolism of FU to FUH_2, the inactive component of FU, with little effect on FUR or FUdR conversion to FU; and 3) thymidine, under certain conditions, appears to prevent the in vivo conversion of FUR and FUdR to FU.

Modulation of antitumor activity by normal metabolites is not restricted to FU. Our results and the data of other researchers (28, 29) have shown that thymidine can also potentiate the toxicity and possibly the antitumor activity of ara-C in rats bearing induced colon carcinoma. Preliminary results seem to indicate that the biochemical basis for the potentiation of ara-C toxicity by thymidine is the dramatic reduction in the circulating CdR pool by thymidine which coincides with the increased uptake and activation of ara-C to the ara-CTP level. These effects were found to be directly related to the steady state level of thymidine achieved during continuous infusion.

Several clinical trials have been initiated to evaluate the efficacy of FU in combination with thymidine against malignancy in patients. In Phase I studies, Woodcock and coworkers (30) demonstrated that prior treatment with thymidine, either 7.5 gm or 15 gm, produces a 10-fold increase in the biological activity of FU when the thymidine is given by rapid infusion and the FU is administered by I.V. bolus injection 60 min following the initiation of the thymidine infusion. The observed toxicity is primarily hematopoietic. Thrombocytopenia was generally more severe than leukopenia. At a dose of 15 gm thymidine and 7.5 mg/kg FU, the median leukocyte nadir was 2,500 as seen on day 17, and the platelet nadir was 97,000 as seen on day 14. After administration of these doses, evidence of antitumor activity was seen in patients with colon and ovarian cancer.

Vogel and coworkers (31) conducted a Phase I study of the combination of FU and thymidine (8 gm/m²/day) by continuous infusion in patients with colon carcinoma. At a FU dose of 7.5 mg/kg/day, gastrointestinal toxicity was minimal and myelosuppression was the dose-limiting factor. Of eight patients with colon carcinoma and no prior chemotherapy, two patients achieved partial responses, and of four patients with prior FU chemotherapy, only one had stable disease. The results of this study, however, indicated that the additon of thymidine to FU by continuous infusion changed the dose-limiting toxicity from gastrointestinal effects to myelosuppression. On the basis of these results, a protocol for evaluation of thymidine in combination with FU by continuous infusion in leukemia patients is underway at the Roswell Park Memorial Institute.

Conclusion

The approach illustrated by the initial studies with ara-C and FU mentioned in this chapter holds promise for future development. Measurement of carefully selected specific biochemical and pharmacological parameters relevant to the action of a specific drug may provide the basis for predicting response in individual patients. Also, it seems logical to assume that differences in the host's metabolism of anticancer drugs contributes significantly to differences in clinical response. These ideas are more readily tested in leukemic patients than in patients with solid tumors, where the technical difficulties of obtaining representative and viable tumor cell suspensions must be added to the general problems related to cell heterogeneity within tumor cell populations. There remains the important task of developing and improving methodologies for obtaining a single and viable cell suspension from solid tumors for the purpose of carrying out biochemical and pharmacological studies.

Modulation of the activities of antimetabolites by normal purine and pyrimidine metabolites have been demonstrated in vitro and in vivo. The mechanism(s) involved and the selectivity of these effects are not yet fully understood. Factors that should be taken into consideration include 1) circulating pools of salvage metabolites in an individual patient before and during therapy, and 2) differential effects and the duration of these effects between normal and tumor tissues. For example, in the subgroup of AML patients in whom the ara-CTP retention is low, it may be possible to increase ara-CTP retention at the target site by administration of a metabolite such as thymidine.

References

1. Grindey, G. B.; Moran, R. G.; and Werkheiser, W. C. Approaches to the rational combination of antimetabolites for cancer chemotherapy. Pp. 169–249 in *Drug design*, vol. 5, ed. E. J. Ariens. New York: Academic Press, Inc., 1975.

2. Mihich, E. et al. UICC workshop on drug resistance and selectivity in cancer chemotherapy. *UICC Technical Report Series* 21:1–37, 1975.

3. Rustum, Y. M. et al. Multifactorial cellular determinants of the action of metabolites. *Adv. Enzyme Regul.* 14:281–295, 1976.

4. Hakala, M. T. Prevention of toxicity of amethopterin for sarcoma-180 cells in tissue culture. *Science* 126:255, 1957.

5. Hakala, M. T., and Taylor, E. The ability of purine and thymine derivatives and of glycine to support the growth of mammalian cells in culture. *J. Biol. Chem.* 234:126–128, 1959.

6. Ensminger, W. et al. Prevention of methotrexate toxicity by thymidine in man. *Proc. Am. Assoc. Cancer Res.* 17:282, 1976.

7. Semon, J. H., and Grindey, G. B. Effect of thymidine on the therapeutic

selectivity of methotrexate in mice. *Proc. Am. Assoc. Cancer Res.* 17:82, 1976.

8. Semon, J. H., and Grindey, G. B. Potentiation of the antitumor activity of methotrexate by concurrent infusion of thymidine. *Cancer Res.* 38:2905–2911, 1978.

9. Kessel, D., and Hall, T. C. Nucleotide formation as a determinant of 5-fluorouracil response in mouse leukemia. *Science* 145:911–913, 1966.

10. Wolberg, W. H. Biochemical approaches to the prediction of response in solid tumors. In Prediction of response in cancer chemotherapy. *Natl. Cancer Inst. Monogr.* 34:189–195, 1971.

11. Klubes, P. et al. Effects of 5-fluorouracil on human colon carcinoma and solid rat Walker 256 carcinoma: evaluation of *in vitro* predictors of clinical response. *Cancer Treat. Rep.* 62:1065–1073, 1978.

12. Rustum, Y. M.; Danhauser, L.; and Wang, G. Selectivity of action of 5-FU: biochemical basis. *Bull. Cancer* (Paris) 66:43–47, 1979.

13. Klubes, P. et al. Effects of 5-fluorouracil on 5-fluorodeoxyuridine-5'-monophosphate and 2-deoxyuridine 5'-monophosphate pools, and DNA synthesis in solid mouse L-1210 and rat Walker 256 tumors. *Cancer Res.* 38:2325–2331, 1978.

14. Ackerman, N. B.; Lien, W. M.; and Silverman, N. A. The blood supply of experimental metastasis III. The effects of acute ligation of the hepatic artery or portal vein. *Surgery* 71:636, 1972.

15. Lien, W. M., and Ackerman, N. B. The blood supply of experimental liver metastasis II. A microcirculatory study of the normal and tumor vessels of the liver with the use of perfused silicone rubber. *Surgery* 68:334, 1970.

16. Suzuki, T. et al. Study of vascularity of tumors of the liver. *Surg. Dev. Oncol.* 134:27, 1972.

17. Yates, J. W. et al. Cytosine arabinoside and daunorubicin therapy in acute nonlymphocytic leukemia. *Cancer Chemother. Rep.* 57:485–489, 1973.

18. Bradey, G. et al. Progress in the treatment of adults with acute leukemia. *Arch. Intern. Med.* 136:1383–1388, 1976.

19. Gale, R. P., and Cline, M. J. High remission induction rate in acute myeloid leukemia. *Lancet* :497–499, 1977.

20. Preisler, H. D. et al. Treatment of acute nonlymphocytic leukemia: use of anthracycline-cytosine arabinoside induction therapy and comparison of two maintenance regimens. *Blood* 53:455–464, 1979.

21. Rustum, Y. M., and Preisler, H. D. Correlation between leukemic cell retention of 1-β-D-arabinofuranosylcytosine 5'-triphosphate and response to therapy. *Cancer Res.* 39:42–49, 1979.

22. Rustum, Y. M. Metabolism and intracellular retention of 1-β-D-arabinofuranosylcytosine as predictors of response of animal tumors. *Cancer Res.* 38:543–549, 1978.

23. Danhauser, L. L., and Rustum, Y. M. A method for continuous drug infusion in unrestrained rats: its application in evaluating the toxicity of 5-fluorouracil/thymidine combinations. *J. Lab. Clin. Med.* 92:1047–1053, 1979.

24. Danhauser, L. L., and Rustum, Y. M. Modification of the toxicity and antitumor activity of 5-fluorouracil (FU) by normal metabolites in rats and mice.

Paper read at the Seventh International Congress of Pharmacology (IUPHAR), 16–21 July 1978, Paris, France.

25. Hakala, M. T., and Rustum, Y. M. The potential value of *in vitro* screening. Pp. 247–287 in *Methods in cancer research*, vol. 16, ed. V. T. DeVita, Jr. and H. Busch. New York: Academic Press, Inc., 1979.

26. Danhauser, L. L., and Rustum, Y. M. Effects of normal metabolites on the efficacy of 5-fluorouracil (FU) against rodents bearing chemically-induced colon tumors. *Proc. Am. Assoc. Cancer Res.* 20:992, 1979.

27. Lee, T.; Rustum, Y. M.; and Bjornsson, S. *In vivo* modulation of the metabolism of fluorinated pyrimidines by normal metabolites, nucleosides and bases. *Proc. Am. Assoc. Cancer Res.* 20:123, 1979.

28. Grant, S.; Goldenberg, I.; and Cadman, E. Augmentation of intracellular cytosine arabinoside accumulation and effect by thymidine in L1210 cells. *Proc. Am. Assoc. Cancer Res.* 20:1046, 1979.

29. Breitman, T. R., and Keene, B. R. Synergistic cytotoxicity to melanomas and leukemias *in vitro* with thymidine and arabinosylcytosine. *Proc. Am. Assoc. Cancer Res.* 20:89, 1979.

30. Woodcock, T. M. et al. Phase I evaluation of thymidine plus fluorouracil (TdR + FU) in patients with advanced cancer. *Proc. Am. Assoc. Cancer Res.* 18:126, 1977.

31. Vogel, S. V. et al. Phase I study of thymidine plus 5-fluorouracil infusion in advanced colorectal carcinoma. *Cancer Treat. Rep.* 63:1–5, 1979.

Chapter 3

The Use of Thymidine to Improve the Therapeutic Selectivity of Antifolates

Gerald B. Grindey, Ph.D.

Introduction

Antifolates have proved to be of major importance in the clinical treatment of cancer since their initial evaluation in 1948 by Farber and coworkers (1). The key role played by dihydrofolate reductase in folate metabolism makes this enzyme a major chemotherapeutic target in the treatment of cancer as well as of several parasitic infections (2). In parasitic infections, the dramatic heterogeneity of dihydrofolate reductase among different species is responsible for a high degree of selectivity with these agents. In the treatment of cancer, however, only a limited degree of selectivity exists, since tumor dihydrofolate reductase is quite similar to the enzyme found in normal cells (3). Because of this restricted selectivity, various approaches have been proposed to improve the therapeutic utility of antifolates; one of these is the combination of methotrexate with thymidine. This chapter will focus only on the basic characteristics of methotrexate and its action which are exploited in pursuing this approach; more comprehensive reviews of the literature on antifolates are currently available (4–13).

Early studies demonstrated the exceedingly tight binding of methotrexate to the target enzyme, dihydrofolate reductase (14, 15), and such binding was termed "stoichiometric" by Werkheiser (14, 15). Inside cells, inhibition of dihydrofolate reductase methotrexate results in a depletion of reduced folate cofactor pools and an increase in the level of dihydrofolate (16, 17). Since cellular maintenance of various tetrahydrofolate cofactors is required for the de novo synthesis of both purines and thymidylate monophosphate (dTMP) (figure 3.1), inhibition of DNA synthesis and consequent cytotoxicity by methotrexate results from disruption of the synthesis of both purine and thymidine deoxyribonucleotide precursors (12). As initially reported by Hakala (18, 19), this inhibition can be prevented in cell culture by supplying the other end products of folate metabolism such as thymidine and hypoxanthine to medium which contains methionine. In most mammalian cells, the addition of either thymidine or hypoxanthine alone is not capable of reversing methotrexate cytotoxicity (12). In certain cells, however, thymidine alone will partially protect cells against the toxic effects of methotrexate (12).

While the mechanism of this partial protection induced by thymidine is not totally understood, one proposal involves the modulation of thymidylate synthetase activity by thymidine-derived increases in the intracellular pool of thymidine 5'-triphosphate (dTTP) (13, 20). As shown in figure 3.1, the synthesis of dTMP by thymidylate synthetase involves the transfer of a 1-carbon unit from a reduced folate cofactor to deoxyuridine monophosphate (dUMP) and the resultant formation of dihydrofolate. Inhibition of dihydrofolate reductase by methotrexate thus interferes with the reduction of dihydrofolate back to tetrahydrofolate, producing a loss of these reduced folate cofactors in the cell. This depletion of reduced folate cofactors would not occur, however, in cells which contained no thymidylate synthetase activity, since this is the only reaction which converts reduced folates to dihydrofolate. Under such conditions no purine toxicity would be expressed, since depletion of the reduced folate cofactor pools would not occur. Thus any agent that modulates thymidylate synthetase activity should alter methotrexate toxicity. Indeed, 5-fluorodeoxyuridine, a potent inhibitor of thymidylate synthetase, was shown to substantially reduce methotrexate toxicity in mice when both agents were administered by continuous infusion (13). Upon metabolic conversion to dTTP, thymidine may decrease the rate of thymidylate synthetase. This decrease may be the consequence of feedback inhibition by dTTP of the pathway of dUMP synthesis (21), resulting in a decrease in intracellular dUMP pools.

Preclinical studies

The ability of thymidine to reduce methotrexate toxicity in vivo was evaluated using a system that allows for long-term continuous I.V. infusion of unrestrained mice (20). In normal DBA/2J mice, the 50% lethal dose of methotrexate infused alone for 48 hr was 6 mg/kg/day. Coadministration of thymidine at 5 gm/kg/day with the methotrexate, followed by an additional 48-hr infusion of thymidine alone, dramatically reduced toxicity. Under these conditions, the 50% lethal dose of

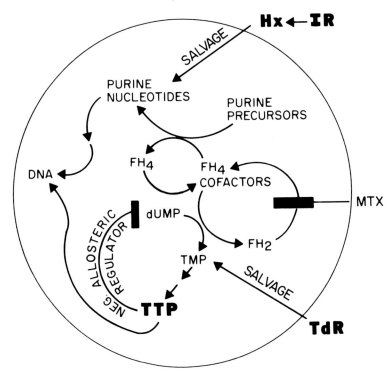

Fig. 3.1   Biochemical pathways involved in the modulation of methotrexate toxicity by thymidine. Abbreviations: IR = inosine, Hx = hypoxanthine, FH_4= tetrahydrofolic acid, FH_2=dihydrofolic acid, dUMP = deoxyuridine-5'-monophosphate, TMP = thymidine-5'-monophosphate, TTP = thymidine-5'-triphosphate, TdR = thymidine, and MTX = methotrexate.

methotrexate was increased sevenfold to about 45 mg/kg/day. In DBA/2J mice bearing leukemia L1210 cells, the infusion of methotrexate alone for 48 hr produced a 33% increase in life span at the optimum dose of 1 mg/kg/day (20). Combination with thymidine resulted in increased therapeutic selectivity, and a 125% increase in life span was obtained with methotrexate at 16 mg/kg/day infused concurrently with thymidine at 5 gm/kg/day (20). The infusion of a source of purine such as inosine, alone or in combination with thymidine, blocked both the toxicity and the antitumor activity of methotrexate. These results indicated that the increase in therapeutic selectivity achieved with the simultaneous infusion of methotrexate and thymidine may result from the complex modulation of the utilization of cellular reduced folates by thymidine as described previously.

Clinical Studies

Although the in vivo results clearly indicate that the therapeutic index of methotrexate in the mouse is improved by the coadministration of thymidine, the implications of extrapolating such results to clinical use are complicated by the effects of the salvage metabolites themselves. In contrast to mouse serum, human serum does not contain xanthine oxidase (22); therefore, the report of the presence of 40 μM hypoxanthine in human serums is not surprising (23). Variation in endogenous purines and other normal metabolites may play a significant role in modulating methotrexate activity against human tumors. Moreover, early reports indicated that the intestine (24) and bone marrow (25) respectively have very low capabilities for de novo purine nucleotide synthesis and may therefore depend primarily on salvageable purines to meet cellular needs. Should this be so, the infusion of thymidine should totally block methotrexate toxicity in intestine and bone marrow tissues. Therapeutic effects, however, might be expected for tumors which require an active de novo pathway to supply cellular purines adequately.

To further evaluate the clinical applicability of these concepts a protocol (26) was designed to accomplish four basic objectives related to improved therapy with high-dose methotrexate:

1. To determine the number of days that high-dose methotrexate can be safely administered in the presence of the concurrent infusion of thymidine
2. To determine whether or not a clinical therapeutic response is possible in the presence of both thymidine and salvageable purines
3. To evaluate whether or not a small amount of leucovorin is also required to stabilize plasma folates during the long-term infusion
4. To determine the therapeutic utility of this new approach with high-dose methotrexate

Twelve patients with various types of metastatic cancer were treated with the methotrexate-thymidine combination as a continuous I.V. infusion (26). Methotrexate was progressively escalated in dose from 2 gm/m²/day for 48 hr to 2 gm/m²/day for 7 days. Concurrently, thymidine at 8 gm/m²/day, together with leucovorin at 1 mg/m²/day, was infused in the same I.V. line and continued beyond the methotrexate infusion until the serum level of drug was less than 2×10^{-8}m. For the 7-day infusions of methotrexate, this usually required an additional 7–10-day infusion of thymidine. Toxicity analysis showed mild mucositis in the majority of cases, and some moderate, reversible bone marrow toxicity (26). Objective antitumor effects were noted in 6 of the 12 patients.

Conclusion

The initial results obtained in human beings indicate that high-dose methotrexate can indeed be administered safely by prolonged infusion in the presence of thymidine. The molecular mechanism for this reversal of toxicity in human beings still is not clearly defined. Results of experiments in mice, however, are consistent with the concept that thymidine modulates the ability of the cell to retain reduced folate cofactors. While the toxicity of methotrexate was dramatically reduced, retention of antitumor activity was demonstrated. The lack of substantial clinical toxicity following a fairly long exposure to high-dose methotrexate may allow this S-phase-specific agent to be of therapeutic use against the more slow-growing solid tumors.

References

1. Farber, S. et al. Temporary remissions in acute leukemia in children produced by folic acid antagonist, 4-aminopteroyl-glutamic acid (aminopterin). *N. Engl. J. Med.* 238:787–793, 1948.

2. Hitchings, G. H. Species differences among dihydrofolate reductases as a basis for chemotherapy. *Postgrad. Med.* (Suppl.) 45:7–18, 1969.

3. Bertino, J. R. Folate antagonists. Pp. 468–483 in *Handbook of experimental pharmacology: antineoplastic and immunosuppressive agents*, vol. 2, ed. A. C. Sartorelli and D. G. Johns. New York: Springer Publishing Co., Inc., 1974.

4. Werkheiser, W. C. Mathematical simulation in chemotherapy. *Ann. NY Acad. Sci.* 186:343–358, 1971.

5. Blakley, R. L., ed., *The biochemistry of folic acid and related pteridines.* New York: Elsevier North-Holland, Inc., 1969.

6. Bertino, J. R., and Johns, D. G. Pp. 9–22 in *Cancer chemotherapy*, vol. 2, ed. I. Brodksy and S. B. Kahn. New York: Grune & Stratton, Inc., 1972.

7. Johns, D. G., and Bertino, J. Pp. 739–754 in *Cancer medicine*, ed. J. F. Holland and E. Frei III. Philadelphia: Lea & Febiger, 1973.

8. Goldman, I. D. Pp. 229–358 in *Drug resistance and selectivity: biochemical and cellular basis*, ed. E. Mihich. New York: Academic Press, Inc., 1973.

9. Hakala, M. T. Pp. 240–263 in *Handbook of experimental pharmacology: antineoplastic and immunosuppressive agents*, vol. 1, ed. A. C. Sartorelli and D. G. Johns. New York: Springer Publishing Co., Inc., 1974.

10. Mead, J. A. R. Pp. 52–71 in *Handbook of experimental pharmacology: antineoplastic and immunosuppressive agents*, vol. 1, ed. A. C. Sartorelli and D. G. Johns. New York: Springer Publishing Co., Inc., 1974.

11. Bertino, J. R. "Rescue" techniques in cancer chemotherapy: use of leucovorin and other rescue agents after methotrexate treatment. *Semin. Oncol.* 4:203–216, 1979.

12. Ensminger, W. D.; Grindey, G. B.; and Hoglind, J.A. Antifolate therapy rescue, selective host protection, and drug combinations. Pp. 61–109 in *Advances*

in cancer chemotherapy, vol. 1, ed. A. Rosowsky. New York: Marcel Dekker, Inc., 1979.

13. Grindey, G. B.; Hoglind, J. A.; and Moran, R. G. Approaches to improved therapeutic selectivity with methotrexate. Pp. 177–190 in *Antimetabolites in biochemistry, biology and medicine,* ed. J. Skoda and P. Langen. New York: Pergamon Press, Inc., 1979.

14. Werkheiser, W. C. Specific binding of 4-amino folic acid analogues by folic acid reductase. *J. Biol. Chem.* 236:888–893, 1961.

15. Werkheiser, W. C. The biochemical, cellular, and pharmacological action and effects of the folic acid antagonists. *Cancer Res.* 23:1277–1285, 1963.

16. Moran, R. G.; Werkheiser, W. C.; and Zakrzewski, S. F. Folate metabolism in mammalian cells in culture. I. Partial characterization of the folate derivatives present in L1210 mouse leukemia cells. *J. Biol. Chem.* 251:3569–3575, 1976.

17. Moran, R. G.; Domin, B. A.; and Zakrzewski, S. F. On the accumulation of polyglutamyl dihydrofolate in methotrexate inhibited L1210 cells. *Proc. Am. Assoc. Cancer Res.* 16:49, 1975.

18. Hakala, M. T. Prevention of toxicity of amethopterin for sarcoma-180 cells in tissue culture. *Science* 126:255, 1957.

19. Hakala, M. T., and Taylor, E. The ability of purine and thymine derivatives and of glycine to support the growth of mammalian cells in culture. *J. Biol. Chem.* 234:126–128, 1959.

20. Hoglind-Semon, J., and Grindey, G. B. Potentiation of the antitumor activity of methotrexate by concurrent infusion of thymidine. *Cancer Res.* 38:2905–2911, 1978.

21. Jackson, R. C. Differential regulation of de novo and salvage pathways of thymidylate biosynthesis in Novikoff hepatoma cells. *Proc. Am. Assoc. Cancer Res.* 19:217, 1978.

22. Al-Khalridi, U. A. S., and Chaglassian, T. H. *The species distribution of xanthine oxidase. Biochem. J.* 97:318–320, 1965.

23. Orsulak, P. T.; Haab, W.; and Appleton, M. D. Quantitative estimation of uric acid, xanthine, and hypoxanthine in plasma using thin-layer chromatography. *Anal. Biochem.* 23:156–162, 1968.

24. MacKinnon, A. M., and Deller, D. J. Purine nucleotide biosynthesis in gastrointestinal mucosa. *Biochim. Biophys. Acta* 319:1–4, 1973.

25. Lajtha, L. G., and Vane, J. R. Dependence of bone marrow cells on the liver for purine supply. *Nature* 182:191–192, 1958.

26. Bruno, S. et al. Methotrexate and thymidine, citrovorum factor in man. *Proc. Am. Assoc. Cancer Res.* 20:434, 1979.

Chapter 4

Human Breast Cancer: Steroid Receptors and Response to Hormonal Manipulation and Cytotoxic Therapy

Fred Rosen, Ph.D.

Introduction

This is an era of intense research into the mechanisms of hormone action. A major part of this effort has been directed toward the characterization and role of receptors in mediating the response of cells to hormones. In the context of steroid hormones, a receptor can be defined as a protein that provides highly specific sites for a steroid in a "target tissue" and, as a consequence of the binding of the steroid to the receptor, the complex formed has the ability to initiate biochemical reactions necessary to produce the end physiological response. A common sequence of steroid-receptor interactions has been observed in target tissues. These include 1) binding of the steroid to a specific cytoplasmic receptor(s), 2) transfer of the steroid-receptor complex from the cytoplasm to the nucleus (temperature dependent), and 3) binding of the complex to specific "acceptor sites" in chromatin (1, 2).

This chapter will focus on the presence of steroid receptors in endocrine-responsive human tumors and their predictive value for therapy. To be selective and critical rather than exhaustive, this chapter will focus on human breast cancer. Within the past decade, mammary carcinoma has been studied extensively with regard to the predictive value of steroid receptors and the correlation of these markers with the tumor's response to hormonal manipulation or treatment with cytotoxic antitumor agents. Therefore, discussion of breast cancer should serve to highlight some of the advances in steroid-receptor research as well as the potential for new therapy of endocrine tumors.

General Principles Governing Steroid-Receptor Interactions

In considering cell membrane receptors for polypeptide or protein hormones, or cytoplasmic and nuclear receptors for the steroid hormones and thyroxine, some general principles apply:

1. The hormone interaction with the receptor should conform to known steric and structural specificity.
2. The binding sites should be finite in number and therefore saturable.
3. Hormone binding should have tissue specificity consistent with biological activity.
4. Hormone binding should be of high affinity (i.e., low dissociation constant) and be observed at physiological concentrations.
5. The binding of the hormone to its receptor should be reversible.

Receptor Assays

In 1960, Jensen and Jacobson (3) reported the synthesis of ^{3}H-estradiol of high specific radioactivity which, when given in physiological doses, was taken up and retained specifically by organs which respond to estrogen treatment. Earlier studies by others, using ^{14}C-labeled steroids of low specific activity, were unsuccessful in demonstrating the presence of estrogen receptors in target tissues. The most important criteria for measuring steroid receptors are 1) the use of ^{3}H-steroids of high specific activity, 2) the need to demonstrate the specificity of the receptor by including a tube with a large excess of the unlabeled steroid or antisteroid, and 3) the recognition that steroid receptors are unstable; therefore, nonequilibrium procedures carried out at low temperatures are required. Three main techniques, gel filtration, charcoal adsorption, and sucrose gradient centrifugation, each of which accomplishes separation of free from bound steroid, are used in this work. The following general procedure was developed by Ip and coworkers (4) for the measurement of cytoplasmic estrogen, progesterone, androgen, and glucocorticoid receptors in normal and malignant tissues, with suitable modifications to correct for binding to the sex steroid binding globulin in human tissue:

1. Tissue is rapidly removed, rinsed in ice-cold saline, trimmed of fat and connective tissue, minced, and homogenized in 6–10 vol of ice-cold TEDG buffer,[1] pH 7.4 at 4°, using a Polytron homogenizer.

---

[1]Tris. buffer, 10 mM; EDTA, 1.5 mM; dithiothreitol, 0.5 mM; glycerol, 10% (v/v).

2. Homogenate is processed in centrifuge for 60 min at 105,000 × g at 4°C supernate (cytosol) is removed; 1 vol dextran-coated charcoal is added to 5 vol cytosol to remove endogenous steroids.
3. Cytosol (75 μl) is incubated with ^{3}H-steroid (10^{-10}–10^{-7}M) in presence or absence of a 100–200-fold molar excess of unlabeled steroid for 2–24 hr at 4°C in microtiter plates.
4. After incubation, bound steroid is removed from free steroid by addition of dextran-coated charcoal (25 μl). It is allowed to stand for 2–10 min, and centrifuged at 850 × g for 10 min at 4°C.
5. An aliquot (70 μl) of supernate is counted in a scintillation counter.
6. "Specific" binding is defined as the difference between total binding and binding in presence of excess unlabeled steroid.

Endocrine Responsiveness of Human Breast Cancer

It is now well established that measurement of the cytoplasmic estrogen receptor can be useful for predicting the response of metastatic breast cancer to hormone manipulation (5, 6, 7). From 75–85% of all primary tumors assayed appear to be positive (> 3 fmoles/mg protein) for the estrogen receptor, of these 55–60% of the patients have been found to respond to endocrine organ ablation (ovariectomy, adrenalectomy, hypophysectomy) or treatment with estrogen or antiestrogens. A number of recent investigations have indicated a correlation between the tumor estrogen receptor level and the disease-free interval, or time of recurrence of malignancy. Patients with estrogen-receptor-positive tumors had longer disease-free intervals than those with tumors that were estrogen-receptor-negative. This relationship held true irrespective of the age of the patient, axillary node status, tumor size, or tumor location (8). Knight and coworkers (9) observed that patients with mammary carcinoma with positive axillary nodes survived significantly longer when the tumor was positive for the estrogen receptor. Positive values can also enable clinicians to predict the longer survival of patients with advanced disease (10).

Estrogen receptor values ranging from 3 to more than 1,000 fmoles/mg protein have been considered to be positive. McGuire and coworkers (8), in a review in which receptor levels were correlated with clinical responsiveness, noted that tumors with high estrogen receptor values (101–1,000 fmoles/mg protein) had a response rate of 81%, whereas only 46% of patients with estrogen receptor values of 3–100 fmoles/mg protein, and 6% of patients with less than 3 fmoles/mg protein responded to endocrine manipulation. Thus the amount of estrogen receptor in a breast tumor, and not merely its presence, is likely to be a more useful value in predicting the likelihood of hormone response.

Correlation Between Positive Estrogen and Progesterone Receptor Values and Endocrine Response in Breast Cancer

It is known that the biosynthesis of the progesterone receptor in guinea pig uterus (11) and breast cancer (12) is regulated by endogenous levels of estrogen or by treatment with this steroid. The induction of the progesterone receptor by estrogen provides a means for determining whether the estrogen receptor is functional. This is especially important in breast cancer, since about 40% of patients with this malignant disease who have positive estrogen receptor values fail to respond to endocrine therapy. Based on these facts, Horwitz and coworkers (13) proposed that measurement of both the estrogen and progesterone receptors in breast cancer would be of greater predictive value for response to endocrine therapy than assay of the estrogen receptor only. Several studies to test this hypothesis have been encouraging (14, 15). In their review, McGuire and coworkers reported that patients positive for estrogen and progesterone show an 83% response rate to endocrine treatment, which compares favorably with the response of patients with high (> 100 fmoles/mg protein) levels of the estrogen receptor and is significantly higher than the 55–60% success rate of hormonal therapy noted in the many studies (8) in which the tumor was considered to be estrogen-receptor-positive (3–1,000 fmoles/mg protein), but was not assayed for the progesterone receptor. It should be noted, however, that the presence of significant amounts of both receptors in a tumor still fails to predict for endocrine response in one out of five patients.

A study by Ip and coworkers (16), using the rat mammary tumor MTW-9B, indicates that there may not always be an association between an estrogen-responsive tumor and progesterone receptor regulation. The MTW-9B tumor contains substantial levels of the estrogen and progesterone receptors, but its growth is unresponsive to ovariectomy or treatment with pharmacological doses of estrogen. Following ovariectomy, the level of the progesterone receptor in the tumor was reduced to 15% of the control value; restoration of this receptor to values seen in intact rats or to higher levels was achieved by treatment with pharmacological doses of estradiol. Thus the estrogen receptor in the MTW-9B tumor is functional for the biosynthesis of the progesterone receptor but is not active in mediating the necessary cellular events which result in an estrogen-responsive mammary tumor. This, then, represents a model system in which the estrogen receptor complex exerts a selective action on the genome, which may explain why a substantial number of patients with an estrogen-receptor-positive tumor, as well as 20% of patients whose tumors contain appreciable amounts of estogen and progesterone receptors, do not respond to endocrine therapy.

Antiestrogen-Induced Remissions in Patients with Breast Cancer

The development of antisteroids preceded the evidence mounted in the mid-sixties that specific cytoplasmic receptors play a key role in mediating the action steroids have on target tissues. Indeed, in their early studies Jensen and coworkers (17) used two antiestrogens, nafoxidine and clomiphene, in competitive binding experiments to demonstrate the specificity of the cytoplasmic rat uterus receptor for 17β-estradiol (Estradiol-17β). Since then, interest in antisteroids has developed because of their potential clinical importance and because studies on their mode of action have provided insight into the complex mechanism by which natural steroids act to stimulate a hormone response. Although antagonists for each steroid are available and currently undergoing evaluation, the antiestrogens have been most extensively investigated, especially with regard to their clinical usefulness in breast cancer therapy.

Two antiestrogens, nafoxidine and tamoxifen, which act by competing with estradiol for the cytoplasmic receptor, have been successful in the treatment of patients with advanced breast cancer (table 4.1). Nafoxidine

Table 4.1 Antiestrogen Treatment of Human Breast Cancer: Response Rate and Estrogen Receptor Correlation

Anti-estrogen	Ref. No.	Dose	Total Responders	Menopausal Status: Responders		Receptor Status: Responders	
				Pre-meno-pausal	Post-meno-pausal*	Estrogen Receptor Positive	Estrogen Receptor Negative
Clomi-phene	(18)	200 or 300 mg/day	19 of 50	0	19 of 50	–	–
Nafoxi-dine	(19)	180–240 mg/day	8 of 23	–	–	8 of 10	0 of 8
Tamoxi-fen	(20)	20 mg × 2/day	24 of 72	1 of 7	23 of 65	11 of 25	0 of 6
Tamoxi-fen	(21)	10 mg × 2/day	16 of 30	1 of 2	15 of 28	8 of 13	0 of 4
Tamoxi-fen	(21)	25 mg × 2/day	19 of 44	1 of 1	18 of 43	–	–

*Natural or ablative.

and tamoxifen have been used to circumvent endocrine ablative procedures such as ovariectomy, adrenalectomy, or hypophysectomy, which have been standard therapy in patients with mammary tumors thought to be dependent on estrogen. This is a notable advance in cancer therapy and provides a strong rationale for the development of antihormones that would be effective against other types of endocrine tumors or certain ectopic tumors that secrete hormones.

Tamoxifen is now widely used in the treatment of postmenopausal women with progressive metastatic breast cancer. The effectiveness of tamoxifen and other antiestrogens in the treatment of these patients is based on the presence of a positive estrogen receptor value; this is because antiestrogens bind tightly to the estrogen receptor and appear to act by inhibiting the expression of the receptor-steroid complex in the nucleus (22, 23).

Various clinical toxicities have been observed in patients on tamoxifen therapy. For the most part, these side-effects have been mild, transient, and dependent on the amount of drug taken. In a typical study, Tormey and coworkers (24) noted a decrease in hemoglobin in patients on low (< 12 mg/m² b.i.d.) compared with patients on higher doses (12–100 mg/m² b.i.d.) of tamoxifen. Interestingly, more instances of leukopenia or thrombocytopenia were observed in patients who received the low dose of tamoxifen. Each of these hematological toxicities reached a peak value by the end of the second week of therapy and, with continued treatment, returned to previous values from 7–12 days later. Because of the transient nature of these effects, it was unnecessary to interrupt therapy in any of the 18 patients studied. Gastrointestinal toxicity, including nausea, vomiting, and distaste for food was encountered in 4 of 18 patients who received a dose of tamoxifen greater than 12 mg/m²; this effect was also observed in other studies (25). Gynecological side-effects of tamoxifen include vaginal discharge and bleeding, and menstrual irregularity.

There are only a few studies on the use of tamoxifen in combination with other steroids or cytotoxic agents. Although it appears that tamoxifen might have an advantage over conventional hormone therapy in the treatment of advanced breast cancer, the results of studies comparing tamoxifen and diethylstilbestrol have not yet been published (26). The results of a clinical trial in which the androgen fluoxymesterone was combined with tamoxifen have indicated that this combination enhanced therapeutic effectiveness (24). The use of the androgen was based on the observation that certain breast tumors that contain androgen receptors are devoid of the estrogen receptor. In these cases, fluoxymesterone might be acting via the androgen or estrogen receptors (27, 28) or indirectly on the pituitary.

Several protocols designed by the European Organization for Research on Treatment of Cancer (EORTC) Breast Cancer Treatment Group have been aimed toward the evaluation of combined hormone (tamoxifen) and cytotoxic therapy for postoperative postmenopausal patients with advanced breast cancer. Heuson (29) reported the results of a trial in which tamoxifen was given continuously at a dose of 20 mg twice daily, and chemotherapy was given concomitantly in two alternate 28-day cycles. In cycle A, adriamycin and vincristine were given, and cycle B involved treatment with cyclophosphamide (Cytoxan), methotrexate, and 5-fluorouracil (FU). Patients were randomly allocated to 12-cycle schedules ABAB and so forth or BABA and so forth. After 1 year (12 cycles), each cycle was extended to 56 days, and doses of the cytotoxic drug were reduced to one-third in patients over age 68. Doses were also reduced in patients with severe toxic reactions. Of the 55 patients in this study that could be evaluated, 13 complete and 27 partical remissions were obtained for an overall remission rate of 73%. Mild to severe toxic side-effects were encountered. These included nausea and vomiting in most of the patients, weakness and pain in two-thirds of the patients, and hematological symptoms in half of the patients. It was concluded that this combination of antiestrogen and cytotoxic chemotherapy represents one of the most effective treatments available for patients with advanced breast cancer.

Cytotoxic Therapy of Advanced Breast Cancer

It has long been known that mastectomy followed by radiotherapy or surgical removal of endocrine glands to suppress the secretion of estrogen does not lead to the cure of metastatic breast cancer. Therefore, investigators turned their attention to the use of adjuvant chemotherapy in patients with advanced disease. Studies of adjuvant therapy (30, 31, 32), begun in the late 1960s, are difficult to evaluate because of lack of controls, differences in patient selection, and the different approach used to treat the local disease. For the most part, these early attempts to treat breast cancer with antitumor agents were unsuccessful, due presumably to the short-term chemotherapy course that was used. Tormey (33) has reviewed these early clinical trials in detail.

A reevaluation of the problem led to the resumption of adjuvant chemotherapy studies in the U.S. in 1972 (34) and in Italy in 1973 (35). These studies differed from the earlier trials in one major facet: based on new observations that some breast cancer cells remain in a nonproliferative state for a long period of time and thus have a long doubling time, chemotherapy was to be started soon after mastectomy and continued for a year or longer. Members of the Eastern Oncology Cooperative Group compared L-phenylalanine nitrogen mustard (L-PAM) with the combination of cyclophosphamide (Cytoxan), methotrexate, and FU (CMF) as adjuvant therapy. In advanced disease, treatment with L-PAM resulted in a 19% response rate that included both complete and partial remission, whereas CMF resulted in a 53% response rate (24, 36, 37, 38).

Subsequently, Bonadonna and coworkers (35) in Milan conducted a study in which postmastectomy patients were randomly assigned to two groups: control (no treatment) or CMF. The results, presented in terms of treatment failure, indicated a significant difference in favor of the CMF-treated patients; this was particularly evident in the patients with four or more positive axillary nodes. In comparison to L-PAM, the advantage of CMF is evident in postmenopausal women, while no difference is seen in premenopausal patients. The reason for this is unknown. The side-effects produced by CMF were more numerous than those seen in patients given L-PAM. CMF treatment was well tolerated, however, as indicated by the fact that an average of 80% of the optimal dose of each drug was administered during the course of the study.

At present, many groups throughout the world are involved in adjuvant chemotherapy treatments for patients who have undergone radical mastectomy and have one or more positive axillary nodes. It will be several years before these new therapies are fully evaluated and their effectiveness compared with L-PAM and CMF.

A number of clinical trials have recently been undertaken to determine whether the level of tumor estrogen receptor was able to predict for response to chemotherapy in metastatic breast cancer. Lippman and coworkers (39) reported that 76% of receptor-poor tumors responded to chemotherapy, whereas only 12% of patients with estrogen-receptor-positive tumors responded. Conversely, Kiang and coworkers (40) observed a significantly higher response to various cytotoxic drug regimens in receptor-rich tumors (86%) than in receptor-poor tumors (36%). In addition, the latter studies revealed no correlation between responses to hormonal therapy and chemotherapy when they were administered sequentially, and attributed this to a possible loss in tumor estrogen receptor during therapy. Mortimer and coworkers (41) also reported that estrogen-receptor-rich tumors responded more favorably to chemotherapy (62%) than did receptor-poor tumors (22%), and concluded that at their clinic, patients positive for the estrogen receptor have a better prognosis and response to chemotherapy then estrogen-receptor-negative patients. In contrast to these results, studies by Rosner and Nemoto (42) and Hilf and coworkers (43) indicated that the response of metastatic breast cancer to chemotherapy was independent of the estrogen receptor status of the tumor.

Conclusion

Steroid hormone receptors in endocrine-responsive tumors provide a determinant for physiological and pharmacological approaches to the treatment of these neoplasms. Indeed, the widespread recognition that the estrogen receptor level predicts for hormone response in breast cancer has already led to significant progress in clinical medicine. Clearly, there is little chance of response to endocrine therapy if the tumor is estrogen-receptor-poor. If the tumor contains ample levels of the estrogen receptor, 55–60% of patients respond to hormone manipulation. This response is increased to 70–80% when both estrogen and progesterone receptors are positive in a tumor. A remaining problem is to identify those patients who are estrogen-receptor-positive and whose tumors have lost hormone dependence, and spare them from ineffective endocrine therapy. The use of steroid hormone receptors to predict for hormonal response of prostate carcinoma and other hormone-sensitive tumors is not as advanced as that for breast cancer. Similarly, the presence of steroid receptors in malignant melanoma (44), renal carcinoma (45, 46), and colon cancer (47) has not been evaluated with regard to the prediction of response to hormonal or cytotoxic therapy.

There is a paucity of information concerning the significance of the presence of androgen and glucocorticoid receptors in breast cancer and the response of the tumor to endocrine organ ablation. In an interesting discussion, Engelsman (48) commented that in premenopausal women the presence of the tumor androgen receptor does not predict for response to estrogen treatment in an estrogen-receptor-positive neoplasm. In four premenopausal women, however, the presence of both androgen and estrogen receptors predicted for response to castration; patients with tumors positive for the estrogen receptor only did not respond. Moreover, when both of these receptors were present in the tumor in adequate levels, the overall remission rate was 75%, whereas when only the estrogen receptor was positive, the remission rate was 56%. In tumors positive for the androgen receptor, but lacking the estrogen receptor, the response to castration was still 44%. Where neither receptor was present, the remission rate was only 4%. While this preliminary report involves only a small number of patients, the results are encouraging and point to new directions in which steroid receptors might be useful in the prediction of endocrine therapy, particularly in premenopausal women.

The response of advanced breast cancer to endocrine therapy appears closely related to the concentration of the estrogen receptor in the tumor. Patients with estrogen receptor values higher than 100 fmoles/mg cytosol protein have a higher remission rate than those who have tumors with lower values. These results are most likely explained in terms of the heterogeneity of cells found in most solid tumors, and the fact that breast tumors are likely to present a mixture of cells, some containing high levels of the estrogen receptor and others devoid of this protein. This probably explains the variation in the magnitude of tumor regression seen in different patients following hormone manipulation, and the fact that regression is never complete and is of limited duration. If we accept the concept that there are variable quantities of estrogen-receptor-negative hormone-insensitive cells in all breast cancers, this could explain the variation in rates of recurrence of the disease that have been noted, as well as development of resistance to hormone therapy. Furthermore, this concept points to the limitation of hormonal therapy and the need to consider cytotoxic agents alone or (preferably) in combination with hormones in an attempt to completely eradicate the disease. The fact that such therapeutic regimens are now being used in many clinics is a most promising development toward the eventual control of metastatic breast cancer.

References

1. Jensen, E. V. et al. A two-step mechanism for the interaction of estradiol with rat uterus. *Proc. Natl. Acad. Sci. USA.* 59:632–638, 1968.

2. Spelsberg, T. C.; Steggles, A. W.; and O'Malley, B. W. Progesterone-binding components of chick oviduct. III. Chromatin acceptor sites. *J. Biol. Chem.* 246:4188–4197, 1971.

3. Jensen, E. V., and Jacobson, H. I. Fate of steroid estrogens in target tissues. Pp. 161–178 in *Biological activities of steroids in relation to cancer,* ed. G. Pincus and E. P. Vollmer. New York: Academic Press, Inc., 1960.

4. Ip, M. M. et al. Characterization of androgen receptors in 7, 12-dimethylbenz(a)anthracene-induced and transplantable rat mammary tumors. *Cancer Res.* 38:2879–2885, 1978.

5. McGuire, W. L.; Carbone, P. P.; and Vollmer, E. P., ed. *Estrogen receptors in human breast cancer.* New York: Raven Press, 1975.

6. McGuire, W. L., ed. Hormones, receptors and breast cancer. In *Progress in cancer research and therapy,* vol. 10. New York: Raven Press, 1978.

7. Heuson, J. C.; Mattheim, W. H.; and Rozencweig, M. *Breast cancer: trends in research and treatment.* European Organization for Research on Treatment of Cancer Monograph Series, vol. 2. New York: Raven Press, 1976.

8. McGuire, W. L., et al. Hormones in breast cancer: update 1978. *Metabolism* (27)4:487–501, 1978.

9. Knight, W. A. et al. Estrogen receptor as an independent prognostic factor for early recurrence in breast cancer. *Cancer Res.* 37:4669–4671, 1977.

10. Walt, A. J. et al. The surgical implications of estrophile protein estimations in carcinoma of the breast. *Surgery* 80:506–512, 1976.

11. Milgrom, E. et al. Mechanisms regulating the concentration and the

conformation of progesterone receptor(s) in the uterus. *J. Biol. Chem.* 248:-6366–6374, 1973.

12. Horwitz, K. B., and McGuire, W. L. Specific progesterone receptors in human breast cancer. *Steroids* 25:497–505, 1975.

13. Horwitz, K. B. et al. Predicting response to endocrine therapy in human breast cancer: a hypothesis. *Science* 189:726–727, 1975.

14. McGuire, W. L. et al. Current status of estrogen and progesterone receptors in breast cancer. *Cancer* 39:2934–2947, 1977.

15. Bloom, N.; Tobin, E.; and Degenshein, G. A. Clinical correlations of endocrine ablation with estrogen and progesterone receptors in advanced breast cancer. Pp. 125–139 in *Progesterone receptors in normal and neoplastic tissue,* ed. W. L. Raynaud and E. E. Baulieu. New York: Raven Press, 1977.

16. Ip, M. M. et al. Mammary cancer: selective action of the estrogen receptor complex. *Science* 203:361–363, 1979.

17. Jensen, E. V. et al. Estrogen receptors and hormone dependency. Pp. 23–58 in *Estrogen target tissues and neoplasia,* ed. T. Dao, Chicago: University of Chicago Press, 1972.

18. Hecker, E. et al. Clinical trial of clomiphene in advanced breast cancer. *Eur. J. Cancer* 10:747–749, 1974.

19. Sasaki, G. H.; Leung, B. S.; and Fletcher, W. S. Therapeutic use of nafoxidine in advanced breast cancer—a correlation with endocrine ablation and tumor estrogen response. *Proc. Am. Soc. Clin. Oncol.* 16:271, 1975.

20. Morgan, L. W., Jr. et al. Therapeutic use of tamoxifen in advanced breast cancer: correlation with biochemical parameters. *Cancer Treat. Rep.* (60)10:1437–1443, 1976.

21. Lerner, H. J. et al. Phase II study of tamoxifen: report of 74 patients with stage IV breast cancer. *Cancer Treat. Rep.* (60)10:1431–1435, 1976.

22. Clark, J. H. et al. Mechanism of action of estogen antagonist: relationship to estrogen receptor binding and hyperestrogenization. Pp. 107–135 in *Hormones, receptors, and breast cancer: progress in cancer research and therapy,* vol. 10. New York: Raven Press, 1978.

23. Katzenellenbogen, B. S. Basic mechanisms of antiestrogen action. Pp. 135–158 in *Hormones, receptors, and breast cancer: progress in cancer research and therapy,* vol. 10. New York: Raven Press, 1978.

24. Tormey, D. C. et al. Evaluation of tamoxifen dose in advanced breast cancer: a progress report. *Cancer Treat. Rep.* (60)10:1451–1459, 1976.

25. Manni, A. et al. Antiestrogen remissions in stage IV breast cancer. *Cancer Treat. Rep.* (60)10:1445–1459, 1976.

26. Roberts, M. M. et al. Preliminary report of a controlled trial in advanced breast cancer comparing tamoxifen with conventional hormone therapy. *Cancer Treat. Rep.* (60)10:1461–1462, 1976.

27. Rochefort, H., and Garcia, M. Androgen on the estrogen receptor. 1. Binding and *in vivo* nuclear translocation. *Steroids* 28:549–560, 1976.

28. Ruh, T. S.; Wassilak, S. G.; and Ruh, M. F. Androgen-induced nuclear accumulation of the estrogen receptor. *Steroids* 25:257–273, 1975.

29. Heuson, J. C. Current overview of EORTC clinical trials with tamoxifen. *Cancer Treat. Rep.* (60)10:1463–1466, 1976.

30. Fisher, B. et al. Surgical adjuvant chemotherapy in cancer of the breast: results of a decade of cooperative investigation. *Ann. Surg.* 168:337–356, 1968.

31. Mansson, B.; Kjellgren, K.; and Nissen-Meyer, R. Cyclophosphamide as adjuvant to the primary surgery for breast cancer, a cooperative controlled clinical study. P. 531 in *Proceedings: 11th International Cancer Congress,* vol. 3. New York: American Elsevier Publishers, Inc., 1974.

32. Rieche, K.; Berndt, H.; and Prahl, B. Continuous postoperative treatment with cyclophosphamide in breast carcinoma: a randomized clinical study. *Arch. Geschwulst-forsch.* 40:349–354, 1972.

33. Tormey, D. C. Combined chemotherapy and surgery in breast cancer: a review. *Cancer* 36:881–892, 1975.

34. Fisher, B. et al. L-Phenylalanine mustard (L-PAM) in the management of primary breast cancer: a report of early findings. *N. Engl. J. Med.* 292:117–122, 1975.

35. Bonadonna, G. et al. Combination chemotherapy as an adjuvant treatment in operable breast cancer. *N.Engl. J. Med.* 294:405–410, 1976.

36. Canellos, G. P. et al. Cyclical combination chemotherapy for advanced breast carcinoma. *Br. Med. J.* 1:218–220, 1974.

37. Taylor, S. G. III et al. Combination chemotherapy for advanced breast cancer: randomized comparison with single drug therapy. P. 175 in *Proceedings: American Association for Cancer Research and American Society for Clinical Oncology Meetings,* vol. 15. Baltimore: Cancer Research, 1974.

38. DeLena, M. et al. Adriamycin plus vincristine compared to and combined with cyclophosphamide, methotrexate, and 5-fluorouracil for advanced breast cancer. *Cancer* 35:1108–1115, 1975.

39. Lippman, M. E. et al. The relation between estrogen receptors and response rate to cytotoxic chemotherapy in metastatic breast cancer. *N. Engl. J. Med.* 298:1223–1228, 1978.

40. Kiang, D. T. et al. Estrogen receptors and responses to chemotherapy and hormonal therapy in advanced breast cancer. *N. Engl. J. Med.* 229:1330–1334, 1978.

41. Mortimer, F. et al. Influence of estrogen receptor (ER) status on survival in metastatic breast cancer. P. 144 in *Proceedings: American Association for Cancer Research and American Society for Clinical Oncology Meetings,* vol. 20. Baltimore: Cancer Research, 1979.

42. Rosner, D., and Nemoto, T. A randomized study of two and three drug regimens in relation with estrogen receptors in metastatic breast cancer. P. 46 in *Proceedings: American Association for Cancer Research and American Society for Clinical Oncology Meetings,* vol. 20. Baltimore: Cancer Research, 1979.

43. Hilf, R. et al. Does estrogen receptor status have prognostic value for recurrence or chemotherapy response in breast cancer? P. 298 in *Proceedings: American Association for Cancer Research and American Society for Clinical Oncology Meetings,* vol. 20. Baltimore: Cancer Research, 1979.

44. Fisher, R. L.; Neifeld, J. P.; and Lippman, M. E. Oestrogen receptors in human malignant melanoma. *Lancet* 2:337–338, 1976.

45. Concolino, G. et al. Progestational therapy in human renal carcinoma and steroid receptors. *J. Steroid Biochem.* 7:923–927, 1976.

46. Bojar, H. et al. Oestrogen-binding components in human renal cell carcinoma. *J. Clin. Chem. Clin. Biochem.* 14:521-526, 1976.

47. Maillot, K. V.; Hermanek, P.; and Gentoch, H. H. Steroid receptors in tumors of tissues generally considered to be hormone-independent. *J. Cancer Res. Clin. Oncol.* 93:77–84, 1979.

48. Engelsman, E. P. 185 in *Breast cancer: trends in research and treatment.* ed. J. C. Heuson, W. H. Mattheiem, and M. Rozencweig. New York: Raven Press, 1976.

Chapter 5

Purine and Pyrimidine Analogs in Cancer Chemotherapy

Alexander Bloch, Ph.D.

Introduction

Among agents of value in the clinical therapy of cancer, purine and pyrimidine analogs play a prominent role. To document this assertion, one need cite only the utility of 6-mercaptopurine (6-MP), 6-thioguanine (6-TG), and cytosine arabinoside (ara-C) in the treatment of various forms of leukemia (1, 2), and the, albeit limited, usefulness of 5-fluorouracil (FU) in the therapy of cancer of the breast, colon, and ovary (3). Since the number of chemical agents of value in current cancer treatment is relatively small, the clinically used purine and pyrimidine analogs constitute a rather significant fraction of these compounds. Thus an introductory overview of the events that have led to the development of these agents and a short review of their biochemical mechanisms of action and clinical usefulness will be presented first.

Development and biochemical effects

6-MP and 6-TG are analogs of the purine bases hypoxanthine and guanine respectively, FU is an analog of uracil, and the nucleoside ara-C can be viewed as an analog of 2'-deoxycytidine. The development of these agents, all of which function as antimetabolites, followed the lead of Domagk (4), Trefouel (5), and Woods (6), who demonstrated in the 1930s that the dye prontosil possesses potent antibacterial effects ascribable to its sulfonamide moiety, which structurally resembles p-aminobenzoic acid, a metabolite required by the affected cells for the synthesis of folic acid.

This lead gave rise to a flurry of activity among chemotherapeutically oriented organic chemists, who began systematically to interchange heteroatoms and functional groups, creating agents that resembled the natural metabolite enough to be activated, but that differed in their function sufficiently to interfere with cell growth. This approach has yielded thousands of analogs of both purines and pyrimidines, and the fact that only a handful of these has shown clinical utility demonstrates that there exist rather stringent requirements concerning the biochemical and pharmacological characteristics that render a compound suitable for therapeutic use (7, 8).

In view of the multiplicity of metabolic sites at which purine analogs can potentially exert their inhibitory effect, identification of the most crucial site of action is not always easy. 6-MP, for instance, has been shown to interfere with the de novo synthesis and interconversion of purine ribonucleotides (9). But 6-MP has also been found to be converted to 6-TG nucleotides and, in this form, to be incorporated into RNA and DNA, the extent of its incorporation into DNA correlating with its cytotoxic effect (10). Similarly, 6-TG, like 6-MP, has been observed to interfere with the de novo synthesis and the interconversion of purine ribonucleotides, but its antitumor effect appears to derive from its incorporation into DNA (11, 12, 13).

Pyrimidine analogs, too, are capable of exerting their effects at multiple sites in the cell metabolism. Ara-C, for example, inhibits nucleotide reductase and DNA polymerase activity in addition to being incorporated into RNA and DNA (14). Similarly, FU is incorporated into RNA and is converted to 5'-fluoro-2'-deoxyuridine-5'-monophosphate, in which form it interferes with the activity of thymidylate synthetase, blocking DNA synthesis by preventing the formation of thymidylic acid (3). Although the direct inhibition of enzymes involved in the biosynthesis of DNA is the metabolic lesion most closely identified with the antitumor action of these two pyrimidine analogs, their incorporation into RNA can affect DNA synthesis indirectly, as is demonstrated by the ara-C-induced inhibition of histone synthesis (15).

Interference with DNA synthesis or function as the crucial step for antitumor activity

What this very brief survey indicates is that, in order to be clinically effective, a purine or a pyrimidine analog may need to interfere primarily with DNA synthesis or function. This suggestion appears to apply to the other clinically useful classes of agents as well. They comprise the alkylating agents, including the various mustards and the nitrosourea derivatives (16–18); the antitumor antibiotics such as daunorubicin (19–20); certain steroid hormones and their analogs (21); and the Vinca alkaloids (22), which interfere with nucleic acid synthesis in addition to inhibiting spindle formation. An exception to this generalization appears to be L-asparaginase, which is thought to deprive sensitive tumor cells of the required amino acid L-asparagine. Although nucleic acid synthesis can be significantly inhibited by the enzyme (23), this effect may be secondary to the inhibition of protein synthesis brought about by the enzyme-induced lack of asparagine. It is to be expected that the temporary deprivation of an amino acid required by the tumor will result in the transient inhibition of its growth without thereby achieving a long-term remission (24). The same transient effect is probably provided by many other cytotoxic agents that are incapable of inducing stable tumor regressions. Indeed, it is remarkable that among the tens of thousands of compounds that have been evaluated, agents that interfere solely with carbohydrate, lipid, or protein metabolism have not demonstrated clinical utility. This fact is probably not ascribable to a lack of differences between tumor and normal cells in the level of enzymes that participate in the activation or metabolism of such analogs. A multitude of data have been accumulated which show that such differences do exist. A compelling conclusion arises from this fact: agents that interfere with DNA metabolism or function produce their therapeutic effects upon tumor cells not merely by inhibiting their growth, but also by effecting changes in the expression of their genetic information, leading to the amelioration of their malignant characteristics. Ample evidence exists to support such a view. A number of laboratories have demonstrated that a variety of antitumor agents which interfere with DNA synthesis or function, and which include 5-bromo-2'-deoxyuridine, 5-fluoro-2'-deoxyuridine, ara-C, adriamycin, and some glucocorticoids, induce myeloid leukemic cells (25), neuroblastoma (26, 27), and erythroleukemia cells (28) to undergo differentiation to mature forms. The possibility must be entertained that long-term remissions are achieved with these agents not only through cell kill, but also through their ability to induce residual tumor cells to reach normal end points.

This postulate implies that cytotoxicity alone is not a good predictor for the antitumor potential of an agent. In fact, as mentioned previously, a great many cytotoxic agents show no selective antitumor effect. What may be necessary for successful clinical activity is cytotoxicity resulting from specific interference with DNA synthesis and/or function that can lead to maturation. Since individual clones of leukemic cells respond differently to various agents, multidrug therapy may be required not only to reduce host toxicity but also to trigger the maturation of the diverse clones of a heterogeneous cell population. Host macrophages may participate in this process, since agents such as poly I-poly C induce them to release factors that stimulate the differentiation of myeloid leukemic cells (29).

Of course, there are on hand a sizable number of purine or pyrimidine analogs, intercalating agents, and alkylators that can modify DNA structure and function without demonstrating antitumor selectivity. The physicochemical properties of these compounds, which result from their structural modifications, clearly determine the extent of their susceptibility to the pharmacological mechanisms operative in the host, including distribution, degradation, and excretion, and thereby contribute to the target selectivity of the agents independently of their capacity to induce differentiation.

Structural and metabolic modulations as means for increasing antitumor effectiveness

At present, it is nearly impossible to predict therapeutic efficacy on the basis of structure alone; therefore, the design of new anticancer agents, including those of the purine and pyrimidine variety, remains an essentially empirical process tempered only by the recognition that some functional groups or some isosteric replacements are more likely to result in favorable biological activity than are others. Since the site of action of therapeutically useful agents is generally the same in tumor and normal cells, structural manipulations that alter their susceptibility to the pharmacological mechanisms of the host constitute a major approach toward improving their selectivity for the tumor. For example, the recently synthesized 2'-azido analog of ara-C, which unlike ara-C is resistant to deamination, is a more effective antileukemic agent than is ara-C, probably as a result of this stability (30).

Protection of host tissues

It is also possible to increase the effectiveness of an antitumor agent through the selective protection of the host tissues from drug-induced toxicity. Use of citrovorum factor or of thymidine for rescue or protection of host tissue from the toxic effects of high doses of methotrexate is a well-established example of this approach (31, 32). Such selective protection extends to nucleoside analogs as well. For instance, testosterone administered to mice up to five days prior to the administration of the antileukemic agent 3-deazauridine markedly reduces the dose-limiting intestinal toxicity of the drug, allowing for its optimum antitumor action (33). More recently, the ability of testosterone to protect the host selectively from FU toxicity has also been reported (34). The intestinal epithelium may be a target tissue for the hormone, and other tissues sensitive to hormonal modulation may be equally amenable to alleviation of drug toxicity by use of this approach, termed "metabolic conditioning" (35).

The clinical utility of purine and pyrimidine analogs can be enhanced by such subterfuges, but it remains to be established whether host protection increases the range of tumors that are sensitive to treatment with the analogs. At present, the purine and pyrimidine analogs are of value for the treatment of leukemias, particularly when used in combination with other agents. Their usefulness for the treatment of solid tumors is rather limited; only FU has elicited some therapeutic responses in cancer of the colon, breast, and ovary. The restricted response of solid tumors is generally ascribed to the limited growth fraction and long cycling time of the small number of proliferating cells. That view neglects the fact that micrometastases of such tumors, which frequently constitute the real clinical problem, may possess a relatively large cycling fraction and yet be insensitive to drug action. One needs to confront the possibility that, unlike the leukemias, the intractable solid tumors cannot be induced to differentiate to mature end points by the chemical agents currently being used, and because complete cell kill is difficult to achieve, permanent tumor regression may not ensue. Consequently, future approaches to the treatment of such tumors may need to employ not only means by which the nongrowth fraction can be induced to enter into cycle (whereupon it would become sensitive to the cytotoxic effects of some currently available drugs), but may also have to make use of agents that can induce the differentiation of malignant cells toward a normal state.

Although extensive experimental exploration is required to establish the practical feasibility of these approaches, they hold promise for the more complete utilization of purine and pyrimidine analogs in future therapy.

References

1. Clarysse, A.; Kenis, Y.; and Mathe, G. Cancer chemotherapy. In *Recent results in cancer research.* New York: Springer-Verlag New York, Inc., 1976.

2. Ho, D.H.W., and Freireich, E. J. Clinical pharmacology of arabinosylcytosine. Pp. 257–271 in *Antineoplastic and immunosuppressive agents II*, ed. A. C. Sartorelli and D. G. Johns. New York: Springer-Verlag New York, Inc., 1975.

3. Heidelberger, C. Fluorinated pyrimidines and their nucleosides. Pp. 193–231 in *Antineoplastic and immunosuppressive agents II*, ed. A. C. Sartorelli and D. G. Johns. New York: Springer-Verlag New York, Inc., 1975.

4. Domagk, G. Ein beitrag zur chemotherapie der bakteriellen infektionen. *Dtsch. Med. Wochenschr.* 61:250–253, 1935.

5. Trefouel, J.; Nitti, F.; and Bovet, D. Activité du p-aminophenylsulfamide sur les infections streptococciques expérimentales de la souris et du lapin. *Soc. Biol.* 120:756–758, 1935.

6. Woods, D. D. The relation of p-aminobenzoic acid to the mechanism of the action of sulphanilamide. *Br. J. Exp. Pathol.* 21:74–90, 1940.

7. Bloch, A. Antimetabolites in cancer chemotherapy. Pp. 163–176 in *Antimetabolites in biochemistry, biology and medicine,* ed. J. Skoda and P. Langen. New York: Pergamon Press, Inc., 1979.

8. Bloch, A. The design of biologically active nucleosides. Pp. 286–360 in *Drug design,* ed. E. J. Ariens. New York: Academic Press, Inc., 1973.

9. Paterson, A. R. P., and Tidd, D. M. 6-Thiopurines. Pp. 384–403 in *Antineoplastic and immunosuppressive agents II,* ed. A. C. Sartorelli and D. G. Johns. New York: Springer-Verlag New York, Inc., 1975.

10. Tidd, D. M. and Paterson, A. R. P. A biochemical mechanism for the delayed cytotoxic effect of 6-mercaptopurine. *Cancer Res.* 34:738–746, 1974.

11. LePage, G. Purine antagonists. Pp. 309–326 in *Cancer. A comprehensive treatise,* vol. 5, ed. F. F. Becker. New York: Plenum Press, 1977.

12. LePage, G., and Whitecar, J. P., Jr. Pharmacology of 6-thioguanine in man. *Cancer Res.* 31:1627–1631, 1971.

13. Nelson, J. A. et al. Mechanisms of action of 6-thioguanine, 6-mercaptopurine and 8-azaguanine. *Cancer Res.* 35:2872–2878, 1975.

14. Creasey, W. A. Arabinosylcytosine. Pp. 232–256 in *Antineoplastic and immunosuppressive agents II,* ed. A. C. Sartorelli and D. G. Johns. New York: Springer-Verlag New York, Inc., 1975.

15. Borun, T. W.; Scharff, M. D.; and Robbins, E. Rapidly labeled, polyribosome-associated RNA having the properties of histone messenger. *Proc. Natl. Acad. Sci. USA* 58:1977–1983, 1967.

16. Ludlum, D. B. Molecular biology of alkylation: an overview. Pp. 6–15 in *Antineoplastic and immunosuppressive agents II,* ed. A. C. Sartorelli and D. G. Johns. New York: Springer-Verlag New York, Inc., 1975.

17. Connors, T. A. Mechanism of action of 2-chloroethylamine derivatives, sulfur mustards, epoxides and aziridines. Pp. 18–30 in *Antineoplastic and immunosuppressive agents II,* ed. A. C. Sartorelli and D. G. Johns. New York: Springer-Verlag New York, Inc., 1975.

18. Wheeler, G. P. Mechanism of action of nitrosoureas. Pp. 65–79 in *Antineoplastic and immunosuppressive agents II,* ed. A. C. Sartorelli and D. G. Johns. New York: Springer-Verlag New York, Inc., 1975.

19. Goldberg, I. H. Actinomycin D. Pp. 582–589 in *Antineoplastic and immunosuppressive agents II,* ed. A. C. Sartorelli and D. G. Johns. New York: Springer-Verlag New York, Inc., 1975.

20. DiMarco, A. Daunomycin (daunorubicin) and adriamycin. Pp. 593–661 in *Antineoplastic and immunosuppressive agents II,* ed. A. C. Sartorelli and D. G. Johns. New York: Springer-Verlag New York, Inc., 1975.

21. Dao, T. L. Pharmacology and clinical utility of hormones in hormone related neoplasms. Pp. 170–188 in *Antineoplastic and immunosuppressive agents*

II, ed. A. C. Sartorelli and D. G. Johns. New York: Springer-Verlag New York, Inc., 1975.

22. Creasey, W. A. Vinca alkaloids and colchicine. Pp. 670–687 in *Antineoplastic and immunosuppressive agents II*, ed. A. C. Sartorelli and D. G. Johns. New York: Springer-Verlag New York, Inc., 1975.

23. Patterson, M. K., Jr. L-asparaginase: basic aspects. Pp. 695–713 in *Antineoplastic and immunosuppressive agents II*, ed. A. C. Sartorelli and D. G. Johns. New York: Springer-Verlag New York, Inc., 1975.

24. Oettgen, H. F. L-asparaginase: current status of clinical evaluation. Pp. 723–742 in *Antineoplastic and immunosuppressive agents II*, ed. A. C. Sartorelli and D. G. Johns. New York: Springer-Verlag New York, Inc., 1975.

25. Sachs, L. Control of normal cell differentiation and the phenotypic reversion of malignancy in myeloid leukaemia. *Nature* 274:535–539, 1978.

26. Schubert, D., and Jacob, F. 5-Bromodeoxyuridine-induced differentiation of a neuroblastoma. *Proc. Natl. Acad Sci. USA* 67:247–254, 1970.

27. Silbert, S. W., and Goldstein, M. N. Drug-induced differentiation of a rat glioma *in vitro*. *Cancer Res.* 32:1422–1427, 1972.

28. Friend, C. et al. Hemoglobin synthesis in murine virus-induced leukemic cells *in vitro*: stimulation of erythroid differentiation by dimethyl sulfoxide. *Proc. Natl. Acad. Sci. USA* 68:378–382, 1971.

29. Tomida, M. et al. Enhancement by double-stranded polyribonucleotides of production by cultured mouse peritoneal macrophages of differentiation-stimulating factor(s) for mouse myeloid leukaemic cells. *Biochem. J.* 176:655–669, 1978.

30. Bobek, M.; Cheng, Y-C.; and Bloch, A. Novel arabinofuranosyl derivatives of cytosine resistant to enzymatic deamination and possessing potent antitumor activity. *J. Med. Chem.* 21:597, 1978.

31. Goldin, A., and Mantel, N. The employment of combinations of drugs in the chemotherapy of neoplasia: a review. *Cancer Res.* 17:635, 1957.

32. Ensminger, W. D.; Grindey, G. B.; and Hoagland, J. A. Antifolate therapy: rescue, selective host protection and drug combinations. Pp. 61–109 in *Advances in cancer chemotherapy*, vol. I, ed. A. Rosowsky. New York: Marcel Dekker, Inc., 1979.

33. Bloch, A. et al. Prevention by testosterone of the intestinal toxicity caused by the antitumor agent 3-deazauridine. *Cancer Res.* 34:1299–1303, 1974.

34. Stolfi, R. L. et al. Protection by testosterone from fluorouracil-induced toxicity without loss of anti-cancer activity against autochthonous murine breast tumors. *Cancer Res.*, 40:2730–2735, 1980.

35. Bloch, A. Metabolic conditioning and metabolic actuation: experimental approaches to cancer chemotherapy involving combinations of metabolites and antimetabolites. *Cancer Chemother. Rep.* 58:471-477, 1974.

Chapter 6

The Regulation
of Ribonucleotide Reductase
and Its Implication
in Cancer Chemotherapy

Yung-Chi Cheng, Ph.D.
and Chi-Hsiung Chang, Ph.D.

Introduction

Ribonucleotide reductase is a key enzyme responsible for the synthesis of all four types of deoxyribonucleotides required for DNA synthesis. Therefore, it has been considered for many years as a target enzyme for anticancer agents. Several deoxyribonucleoside analogs such as arabinosyladenine, cytosine arabinoside (ara-C), 5-fluoro-2'-deoxyuridine, and iododeoxyuridine are used currently in clinics for the treatment of cancer or virus-induced diseases. The action of these analogs depends on the extent of their activation and catabolism in target cells as well as on the size of the pools of deoxyribonucleotides which could interfere with drug metabolism or compete with and/or reverse their effects. The pool sizes of deoxyribonucleotide are to a certain extent regulated by the activity of ribonucleotide reductase. Thus regulation of ribonucleotide reductase in cells could affect the potency of deoxynucleoside analogs as anticancer or antivirus agents. In order to explore the regulation of ribonucleotide reductase, it is essential to understand its properties.

Enzyme properties and activity

While ribonucleotide reductase obtained from bacterial sources (1–6) has been purified and well characterized, the properties of the enzyme obtained from mammalian cells have not been completely described due to difficulties in purification, although some properties of the partially purified enzyme derived from mammalian sources have been reported

(7–11). For the past few years, we have concentrated our efforts in purifying ribonucleotide reductase derived from human sources. In addition, using a highly purified preparation, we have examined some properties of this enzyme. The results obtained in our laboratory may provide new leads for the development of anticancer agents and are discussed in this chapter.

It has been proposed that in mammalian cells there are different enzymes responsible for the reductions of adenosine 5'-diphosphate (ADP) and cytidine diphosphate choline (CDP) (9, 12, 13). This proposal is based on the observation that ADP and CDP reductase activities fluctuate independently throughout the cell cycle in Chinese hamster cells (12) or in regenerating rat liver (13).

We examined the enzymatic reduction of ADP and CDP at different stages of the cell cycle in HeLa cells synchronized by the mitotic selection technique (14). There was no detectable enzyme activity for CDP and ADP reduction in cells in the G_1 phase, and both enzyme activities began to increase and reached a peak in early S phase. The enzyme activity then decreased sharply as the cells entered mitosis. The rate of reduction of ADP and CDP fluctuated in a similar manner throughout the cell cycle. Thus there was no indication of separation of the enzymatic reduction of these substrates. Another piece of evidence supporting the concept of the existence of two separate enzyme entities for the reduction of CDP and ADP in mammalian cells is based on the observation that ADP and CDP reductase activities derived from mouse ascites cells are affected differently by various inhibitory agents. This observation could be simply explained, however, by proposing two different configurations of the active site involved in ADP and CDP reduction.

Isolation from human cell lines

In order to further establish that reduction of ribonucleotides is catalyzed by the same enzyme, we extensively purified ribonucleotide reductase from a human cell line (MOLT-4F) grown in cell culture (15). There was no dissociation of CDP and ADP reductase activities throughout the entire purification process. The purified enzyme preparation reduced all four ribonucleoside 5'-diphosphates: ADP, guanosine 5'-diphosphate (GDP), CDP, and uridine diphosphate (UDP). This result supports the concept that one enzyme entity is responsible for the reduction of the four ribonucleoside diphosphates in the MOLT-4F human cell line. Therefore, an inhibitor for ribonucleotide reductase could possibly be devised that would inhibit the synthesis of all four deoxyribonucleotides.

In order to find out whether ribonucleotide reductase derived from one type of human cells may differ from enzyme obtained from other types of human cells, the behavior of ribonucleotide reductase derived from several different human cell lines in culture and from tumor cells obtained from patients was examined.

On the basis of their behavior upon ammonium sulfate fractionation, two groups of ribonucleotide reductase were identified. The enzyme found in KB, Connaughton, or histocytic lymphoma cells (group I) was precipitated in the 0–35% ammonium sulfate fraction, whereas the enzyme activity derived from MOLT-4F or HeLa-S3 cells (group II) was precipitated in the 35–50% ammonium sulfate fraction (16). The enzyme derived from group I had a different sedimentation rate than that of group II. In addition, these groups of enzymes exhibit different responses to agents such as hydroxyurea, 1-formyl-isoquinoline thiosemicarbazone (IQ-1), and 1,10-phenanthroline. It should be emphasized that both CDP and ADP reductase activities from both groups cosedimented in ammonium sulfate fractionation and sucrose gradient centrifugation. Thus it can be concluded that the ribonucleotide reductase derived from one human cell line can be different from that derived from another human cell line.

The observation of the heterogeneity of enzyme derived from different human cell lines raises the possibility that different isozymes may exist in different tissues, and hence that some tumor cells may possess a different isozyme from that present in normal cells. Can an anticancer agent be developed on the basis of differences in ribonucleotide reductase in tumor and normal cells? In order to answer this question, we have purified and examined the properties of the enzyme. So far, we have obtained highly purified enzyme derived from the MOLT-4F cell, a T-type human lymphoblast cell originally derived from acute lymphocytic leukemia by Dr. Minowada of the Roswell Park Memorial Institute (15).

Ribonucleotide reductase from MOLT-4F cells was found to be composed of two components that were dissociated by deoxyguanosine 5′-triphosphate (dGTP)-sepharose column chromatography. These components were then further purified by DEAE-cellulose, blue-sepharose, and phenyl-sepharose column chromatography. Both components are required to give the enzyme activity; neither by itself has any known catalytic activity. The reconstituted enzyme from the two highly purified components does not require exogenous addition of ferrous or ferric ion for its activity, but magnesium ion is required for activity.

Polyamines can be substituted for magnesium in the reduction of CDP but not in that of ADP. This observation implies that polyamines may be involved in the regulation of deoxyribonucleotide metabolism in human cells. Therefore, a chemotherapeutic agent designed to interfere with polyamine metabolism may also lead to disturbances in deoxyribonucleotide metabolism.

The kinetic behavior of reconstituted enzyme from MOLT-4F cells was examined. It was found (17–19) that adenosine 5'-triphosphate (ATP) has different effects on all forms of ribonucleotide reduction. ATP can activate both CDP and UDP reduction, with an apparent K_a value of 0.63 ± 0.03 and 1.25 ± 0.10 mM respectively. It appears to exert its activation by enhancing the binding affinity of CDP or UDP for the enzyme (19). Guanosine 5'-triphosphate (GTP) or dGTP, but not ATP, activated the reduction of ADP with a K_a value of 1.1 mM for both; and deoxythymidine 5'-triphoshate (dTTP), but not ATP, activated reduction of the ADP with a K_a value of 1.3 μM. The binding affinity of GTP or dGTP for the enzyme, however, was enhanced by ATP about 10 fold, and the maximum velocity of dTTP-activated GDP reduction was increased fourfold in the presence of ATP. In general, the activator for each ribonucleotide reduction seems to enhance the binding affinity of the substrate to enzyme. Because ATP plays a key role in all four reductions, this implies that the intracellular energy charge plays a role in the regulation of ribonucleotide reductase activity. Thus an interference with carbohydrate metabolism in cells could lead to the regulation of ribonucleotide reductase activity.

Ribonucleotide reductase is affected by various nucleotides. The reduction of each ribonucleoside diphosphate can be affected by other ribonucleoside diphosphates and triphosphates. Therefore, imbalances in the physiological concentration of ribonucleotides could change the intracellular concentration of deoxyribonucleotides. Deoxyribonucleotides could also affect ribonucleotide reductase. Deoxyadenosine 5'-triphosphate (dATP) acts as a noncompetitive inhibitor with respect to either activator or substrate. The K_i slope was equal to K_i intercept in the reduction of ribonucleoside diphosphates when the reaction was examined with limited amounts of activator and excess amounts of substrates. This implies that the activator will not interfere with the binding of dATP.

The K_i slope and K_i intercept are different, however, when the reaction is examined against variable amounts of substrate and an excess amount of activator. This implies that nucleoside diphosphates may affect the binding of the inhibitor, dATP, to the enzyme (18). Ara-ATP, an analog of dATP, is also an inhibitor of CDP and ADP reduction. Examination of the effects of ara-ATP on UDP and GDP reduction is still in progress. dGTP, not GTP, acts as a potent inhibitor of UDP and CDP reduction. This implies that dGTP may have a site in addition to GTP for the enzyme, and furthermore that this additional site may be different from the dATP binding sites.

So far, all the results obtained indicate that ribonucleotide reductase is highly regulated by the steady state intracellular concentrations of all the nucleotides. Therefore, a perturbation of the pool size of nucleotides, whether deoxy- or ribonucleotides, could lead to changes in reduction of the ribonucleoside diphosphates. Thus it may be possible to modulate the regulation of ribonucleotide reductase activity by altering the intracellular nucleotide pools.

As is indicated in this brief discussion, the study of the activity and regulation of a key enzyme along the biosynthetic pathways leading to the formation of DNA may provide not only important information on basic aspects of cell metabolism, but may also yield important leads which may ultimately result in the formulation of new cancer therapies. It may be possible to develop inhibitors of ribonucleotide reductase that affect enzyme activity in some tumor cells but not in other cells; modification of polyamine metabolism by drugs may affect the regulation of this enzyme. Drug interference with adenylate charge may modulate the activity of ribonucleotide reductase. In general, modifications of ribonucleotide and deoxynucleotide pools through pharmacological means may modulate selectively the activity of ribonucleotide reductase in target cancer cells but not in normal tissues.

References

1. Brown, N. C. et al. Ribonucleoside diphosphate reductase. Purification of the two subunits, proteins B1 and B2. *Eur. J. Biochem.* 9:561–573, 1969.

2. Holmgren, A.; Reichard, P.; and Thelander, L. Enzymatic synthesis of deoxyribonucleotides, VIII. The effects of ATP and dATP in the CDP reductase system from *E. coli. Proc. Natl. Acad. Sci. USA.* 54:830–836, 1965.

3. Thelander, L. Reaction mechanism of ribonucleoside diphosphate reductase from *Escherichia coli. J. Biol. Chem.* 249:4858–4862, 1974.

4. Brown, N. C. Spectrum and iron content of protein B2 from ribonucleoside diphosphate reductase. *Eur. J. Biochem.* 9:512–518, 1969.

5. Goulian, M., and Beck, W. S. Purification and properties of cobamide-dependent ribonucleotide reductase from *Lactobacillus leichmannii. J. Biol. Chem.* 241:4233–4242, 1966.

6. Vitols, E. et al. Cobamides and ribonucleotide reduction. *J. Biol. Chem.* 242:3035–3041, 1967.

7. Moore, E. C. Mammalian ribonucleoside diphosphate reductase. Pp. 155–164 in *Methods in enzymology,* vol. 12, part A, ed. L. Grossman and K. Moldave. New York: Academic Press, Inc., 1967.

8. Moore, E. C. Components and control of ribonucleotide reductase system of the rat. Pp. 101–114 in *Advances in enzyme regulation,* vol. 15, ed. G. Weber. New York: Pergamon Press, Inc., 1976.

9. Cory, J. G.; Mansell, M. M.; and Whitford, J. W., Jr. Control of ribonucleotide reductase in mammalian cells. Pp. 45–62 in *Advances in enzyme regulation,* vol. 14, ed. G. Weber. New York: Pergamon Press, Inc., 1975.

10. Hopper, S. Ribonucleotide reductase of rabbit bone marrow: I. Purification, properties, and separation into two protein fractions. *J. Biol. Chem.* 247: 3336–3340, 1972.

11. Larsson, A. Ribonucleotide reductase from regenerating rat liver. *Eur. J. Biochem.* 11:113–121, 1969.

12. Peterson, M. D., and Moore, E. C. Independent fluctuations of cytidine and adenosine diphosphate reductase activities in cultured Chinese hamster fibroblasts. *Biochim. Biophys. Acta* 432:80–91, 1976.

13. Collins, T.; David, F.; and Van Lancker, J. L. CDP and ADP reductase in rat regenerating liver. *Fed. Proc.* 31:641, 1972.

14. Cheng, Y-C. et al. Fluctuations of ribonucleotide reductase activity and deoxyribonucleotide pools in synchronized HeLa cells. *Proc. Am. Assoc. Cancer Res.* 18:185, 1977.

15. Chang, C-H., and Cheng, Y-C. Demonstration of two components and association of adenosine diphosphate-cytidine diphosphate reductase from cultured human lymphoblast cells (MOLT-4F). *Cancer Res.* 39:436–442, 1979.

16. Chang, C-H., and Cheng, Y-C. Ribonucleotide reductase isolated from human cells: I. Heterogeneity among the sources. *Biochem. Pharmacol.* 27:2297–2300, 1978.

17. Chang, C-H., and Cheng, Y-C. Properties of ribonucleotide reductase isolated from a human lymphoblast line (MOLT 4F). *Proc. Am. Assoc. Cancer Res.* 19:271, 1978.

18. Chang, C-H., and Cheng, Y-C. Kinetic behavior of ribonucleotide reductase from human MOLT-4F cells. *Fed. Proc.* 38:484, 1979.

19. Chang, C-H., and Cheng, Y-C. Substrate specificity of human ribonucleotide reductase from MOLT 4F cells. *Cancer Res.* 39:5081–5086, 1979.

Chapter 7

Membrane Metabolism as a Target in Cancer Chemotherapy

Ralph J. Bernacki, Ph.D.
and Michael J. Morin, Ph.D.

Introduction

The cell surface is known to play a significant role in many of the cell's biological processes. The importance of the cell surface in cell growth, transport, division, cell-to-cell communication, movement, and differentiation, as well as its impact on other diverse physiological phenomena is now well recognized (1). Alterations in any of these parameters may lead to a loss of growth control and malignancy (2). Many reports have appeared showing differences in the morphological characteristics and biochemical composition of the cell surface following neoplastic transformation. Transformed cells generally exhibit 1) loss of density-dependent inhibition of movement and growth, 2) loss of high molecular weight large external transformation-sensitive (LETS) plasma membrane protein (3), 3) decreased growth dependence on serum, 4) increased ability to grow in semisolid medium, 5) increased lectin agglutinability, 6) changes in antigenic components, 7) altered glycosylation of membrane proteins and lipids, and 8) decreases in the level of membrane adenylcyclase (4). Since these membrane properties are altered in neoplastic cells, it may follow that surface modifications are related to and perhaps even instrumental in neoplastic cell behavior. Therefore, the plasma membrane of the tumor cell may be a unique target for cancer chemotherapy which has not been fully exploited.

A variety of approaches that use the cell membrane as a target for cancer chemotherapy are currently being evaluated. The membrane-active agents that have some chemotherapeutic potential are

The agents outlined can be divided into two basic groups. One is based upon direct membrane modifications caused by lipophilic agents, and the other is based upon interference or alteration in membrane glycoconjugate biosynthesis. The agents in both groups may cause alterations of membrane structure that result in changes in membrane permeability, increases in cellular immunogenicity, or changes in other cellular membrane properties. These changes may alter cellular behavior and the malignant potential of tumor cells.

Lipophilic Agents Displaying Chemotherapeutic Potential

Liposomes

Liposomes, unilamellar phospholipid vesicles of various sizes and compositions, are currently being evaluated for their ability to act as drug depots or carriers potentially capable of targeting cytotoxic agents to specific loci (5–7). Liposomes may also circumvent decreased drug uptake in drug-resistant cells by transferring their contents directly to cells by fusion with the cell's plasma membranes. This was observed to occur in vitro when transport-resistant cells were exposed to liposomes containing actinomycin D. RNA synthesis and cell growth was inhibited under these conditions (8). Uptake of liposomes administered occurred principally in the liver and spleen (9). Even though most liposomes are cleared by the reticuloendothelial system, increased survival times have been observed in L1210-tumor-bearing mice receiving liposomes containing arabinofuranosylcytosine (10). This response was due presumably to depot formation and sustained release of drug. Local hyperthermia of subcutaneous Lewis lung tumor cells combined with the administration of methotrexate containing liposomes resulted in increased uptake of the drug into tumor cells. This increase was caused by increased efflux of the drug from the liposomes in heated tissues (11). Targeting of liposomes to specific tumor sites is the next goal of a number of laboratories, but at this time little success has been reported.

Anthracycline Antibiotics

Many of the nucleic acid intercalators such as the anthracycline antibiotics (i.e., adriamycin) and the diacridines may owe their selective tumoricidal effects to their ability to interact with tumor plasma membrane components in addition to their binding to nucleic acids. Adriamycin has been shown to increase the rate of agglutination of sarcoma 180 (S180) cells by concanavalin A (12) and to increase the phase transition temperature of phospholipid membranes containing cardiolipin (13). Diacridines and actinomycin have been shown to decrease the rate of agglutination of S180 or P388 tumor cells induced by concanavalin A or wheat germ agglutinin respectively. An inverse correlation between the survival times of animals bearing these tumors and the rates of cellular agglutination following treatment with these drugs was also noted (14). Therefore, one can conclude that the chemotherapeutic potential of these agents may be somehow related to a membrane-mediated effect and that this effect is related to lectin-induced agglutination.

Porphyrins

Another lipophilic agent owing some of its chemotherapeutic activity to its affinity with plasma membrane is porphyrin. The initial site of action of the photoactivated porphyrins is at the cell membrane (15). The first characteristic of the action of these compounds is their lipid solubility. Porphyrins with high octanol/water partition coefficients are most cytotoxic. Therefore, plasma membrane is the initial site of action for these compounds.

Polyene Antibiotics

The polyene antibiotics are another example of lipophilic chemotherapeutic agents owing their effectiveness to their interactions with plasma membrane. Amphotericin B is known to interact with sterol components of cell surfaces, thereby altering membrane permeability.

Medoff and coworkers (16) found that combining amphotericin B with an alkylating agent resulted in a synergistic chemotherapeutic response. This enhanced effect may have been due in part to increased permeability of the tumor cells to the alkylating agent. Alternatively, the synergistic response may have been a result of alterations in cell surface antigenicity leading to increased cellular immunogenicity.

Glycoconjugate Modifiers Exhibiting Chemotherapeutic Potential

Neuraminidase

Immunotherapy involving membrane alteration was pioneered by Bekesi and coworkers (17) and Simmons and Rios (18), who used bacterial neuraminidase to treat tumor cells. Neuraminidase, a glycosidase obtained from *Vibrio cholerae,* has been used to remove terminal sialic acids from the surface glycoconjugate of tumor cells. This treatment has been shown to decrease the electrophoretic mobility of cells and to "unmask" certain antigenic sites on these cells. Some therapeutic success has been obtained in animal tumor systems and in patients with acute myelocytic leukemia (AML) following the inoculation of neuraminidase-treated tumor cells. Patient immunization was effected by intradermal injections, at 50 different sites, of approximately 1.5×10^8 neuraminidase-treated allogeneic AML cells per site. At 48 hr, reaction to the neuraminidase-treated cells was measured by induration at the injection site. Biopsies of cutaneous reaction sites showed immunoblastic infiltration. In a limited study of 10 patients who had relapsed from previous antileukemic therapy and who were reinduced, 6 immunized patients had remission durations more than twice the length of the controls. In previously untreated patients, the median remission duration for 7 patients on chemotherapy alone was 20 weeks, while 5 of 7 patients receiving neuraminidase-treated allogeneic myeloblasts remained in remission for 68–112 weeks (19). Larger clinical studies are currently under way.

L-Asparaginase

L-Asparaginase, an enzyme that catalyzes the hydrolysis of asparagine to aspartic acid, has been shown to be an effective chemotherapeutic agent for the treatment of human leukemia. Certain neoplastic tissues have an essential requirement for the amino acid asparagine, while most normal tissues synthesize their own supply (20). Asparagine is also essential for the biosynthesis of glycoprotein. The initial attachment of sugar to protein is mediated in many cases by an N-glycosidic linkage between N-acetylglucosamine and asparagine residues. Bosmann and Kessel (21, 22) have shown that L-asparaginase inhibits the incorporation of labeled L-fucose and D-glucosamine into glycoprotein of L5178Y murine leukemia cells. This effect is probably related to the inhibition of protein synthesis, although the inhibition of glycoprotein synthesis occurred earlier than the inhibition of protein synthesis. The inhibition of sugar incorporation may be related to the rapid dissolution of membranes also observed with L-asparaginase (23).

Sugar Analogs

The biosynthesis of plasma membrane glycoconjugates presents a number of enzymatic sites for interaction with potential antitumor agents (fig. 7.1). Mammalian cells are capable of synthesizing all their membrane carbohydrate from glucose but are capable of using exogenous membrane sugars as well. These sugars are phosphorylated by various kinases and later conjugated with nucleotides to form nucleotide-sugars. The nucleotide-sugars act as substrates for a variety of glycosyl transferases which covalently attach these sugars to form glyconjugate (24). The enzymatic activity of these glycosyl transferases is partially regulated by nucleotide pools (25) and by the availability of substrates and other cofactors.

In the past nine years, evidence has accumulated that indicates that assembly of oligosaccharide chains of glycoprotein is a complex process that involves the participation of lipid intermediates such as dolichol (26) and retinol (27). Dolichol has been implicated in the transfer of the innermost core sugars to asparagine via an N-glycosidic linkage (an alkali-stable bond); retinol has been implicated as a donor of sugars to protein, forming an alkali-labile linkage, presumably an O-glycosidic bond with serine or threonine. Several antibiotics have been found to interfere with lipid-mediated glycoconjugate biosynthesis (i.e., tunicamycin) and these compounds may have some potential as cancer chemotherapeutic agents.

In the past few years, our laboratory at the Grace Cancer Drug Center has focused on the design and evaluation of several sugar analogs and nucleotide-sugar analogs synthesized by Dr. W. Korytnyk, and of tunicamycin, provided by Eli Lilly and Company, as potential cancer chemotherapeutic agents.

Analogs of glucosamine, galactosamine, galactose, mannose, fucose, and sialic acid have been synthesized (28–30) and tested (31, 32) in a number of experimental systems for their chemotherapeutic potential. The following is an outline of the biological test systems used in the assessment of carbohydrate analog activity:

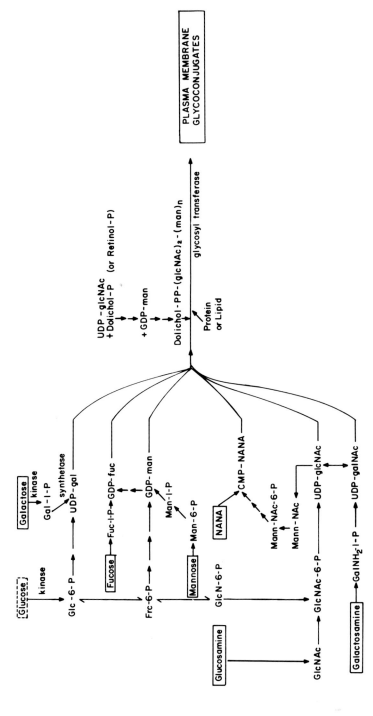

Fig. 7.1 Biosynthesis of plasma membrane glycoconjugate (a simplified scheme). Dotted lines around glucose indicate de novo pathways while the solid lines around the other sugars indicate salvage pathways that might be affected by simple sugar analogs.

I. In vitro systems
  A. Cytotoxicity tests (establishment of inhibitory concentration, or IC_{50} values) (30–32)
  B. Incorporation studies (30–32)
  C. Electron microscope localization studies (32)
  D. Effects on ribonucleotide pool sizes and combination chemotherapy studies (32)
  E. Inhibition of sialyltransferase activity by nucleotide or nucleotide-sugar analogs (32, 33)
II. In vivo systems
  A. Percentage of increase in life span of L1210-tumor-bearing animals (32, 34)
  B. Transplantability of leukemia (35)

Growth-inhibitory concentrations for all analogs are established with L1210 leukemic cells maintained in vitro. Basically, L1210 cells are grown in Roswell Park Memorial Institute (RPMI) 1640 plus 10% fetal calf serum for 42 hr in the presence of various concentrations of the analogs. Cell growth is monitored with a Coulter counter and expressed as the percentage of control growth. These data are plotted, and the concentration of agent necessary to inhibit growth by 50% (IC_{50} is calculated (fig. 7.2).

The acetylation of glucosamine to form 2-acetamido-2-deoxy-1, 3, 4, 6-tetra-O-acetyl-β-D-glucopyranose, or simply β-penta acetylglucosamine (β-PAG), resulted in a compound with increased cytotoxic potential (31). The IC_{50} for glucosamine was 9.0 mM and that for β-PAG 0.33 mM. This increase in cytotoxicity may be a result of the increased lipid solubility of β-PAG; the octanol/water partition coefficient for β-PAG was 0.424, while glucosamine was not readily soluble in octanol (31). Both compounds effectively decreased intracellular uridine triphosphate (UTP) pools via the formation of large amounts of nucleotide-sugar (31), but neither of these compounds have shown any chemotherapeutic activity in vivo against L1210 leukemia in DBA/2 female mice.

Azaribine, a uridine analog that inhibits orotidylate (OMP) decarboxylase (36) and blocks de novo synthesis of uridylate, had an IC_{50} of 1.9×10^{-6}M (fig. 7.2). This compound has been combined with glucosamine and β-PAG to enhance the cytotoxic effects of the sugar and sugar analog.

Combination Chemotherapy Using Sugars and Nucleoside Analogs

The use of combinations of membrane sugars or sugar analogs with nucleoside analogs has resulted in increased cytotoxicity and in some cases synergistic effects in vitro (37, 38). We have investigated the effects of

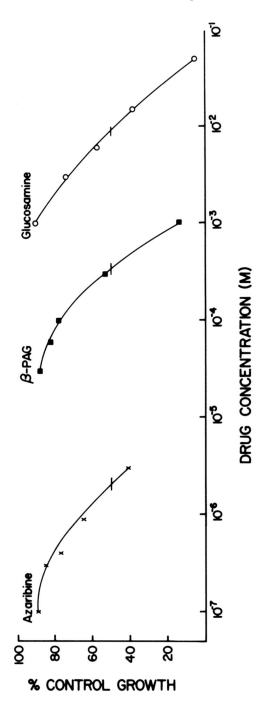

Fig. 7.2 Effects of azaribine, β-penta acetylated glucosamine (β-PAG) and glucosamine on L1210 murine leukemia growth in vitro.   Bars (—) indicate IC_{50} concentrations.

combinations of galactosamine, glucosamine, and β-PAG with either 3-deazauridine (DAUR) or azaribine (an acetylated derivative of 6-azauridine) on the growth and ribonucleotide pool sizes of L1210 murine leukemia cells in vitro. The combination of amino sugars with DAUR resulted in antagonistic drug interactions in both L1210 cells and human HeLa cells (32). This was due to a lowering of cytotoxic DAUR-metabolite, 3-deaza UTP (fig. 7.3), which inhibits the formation of cytidine triphosphate (CTP) from UTP by blocking CTP synthetase (39).

L1210 cells were incubated in 10 ml RPMI 1640 plus 10% fetal calf serum plus 0, 1, 5, and 10 mM glucosamine for 24 hr. [^{3}H]-DAUR (5 μCI) was added to each culture 1 hr after the addition of glucosamine. Twenty-four hours later, 10^7 cells were extracted with 6% perchloric acid (100 μl/10^7 cells) and 10 μl of the acid-soluble fraction was analyzed for its [^{3}H]-deazauridine ribonucleotide content using a Dupont 830 high-pressure liquid chromatographic system (40). Fractions (1.5 min, 0.7 m l) were collected from the column and counted in Aqueous Counting Scintillant using a Packard liquid scintillation counter. Four peaks of radioactivity were observed which correspond to deazauridine monophosphate (deaza-UMP), deazauridine diphosphate (deaza-UDP), deaza-UDP-sugar, and deazauridine triphosphate (deaza-UTP) (fig. 7.3). The amount of deaza-UTP is highest in control cells, with the most abundant peak-4 fraction containing 1,750 c.p.m. The addition of glucosamine to the cultures resulted in a decrease of deaza-UTP content to 1,050 c.p.m. (at 10mM glucosamine) and an increase in peak-2 deaza-UDP-sugar. The formation of deaza-UDP-sugar resulted in a lowering of deaza-UTP levels either directly or indirectly, which may account for the pharmacological antagonism evident with this combination of agents in L1210 and HeLa cells (32). Jackson, Williams, and Weber (32) found that a combination of DAUR with galactosamine resulted in additive pharmacological effects with a different subline of L1210 leukemia cells, while this combination of agents had synergistic effects against a number of hepatoma cell lines. Minimal-deviation hepatomas were more susceptible to this therapy than more dedifferentiated hepatomas. The differences in response to a combination of DAUR and amino sugar reflect differences in intracellular metabolism and cell type.

In our laboratory, the addition of azaribine with glucosamine or β-PAG to L1210 cells resulted in pharmacologically additive or synergistic effects, depending on whether the agents were added simultaneously or sequentially. Cultures of L1210 cells were incubated in 1 ml RPMI-1640 plus 10% fetal calf serum containing azaribine and glucosamine or β-PAG at or near their IC_{50} concentrations. The agents were added either simultaneously (figs. 7.4 and 7.5) or sequentially (figs. 7.6 and 7.7). The simultaneous

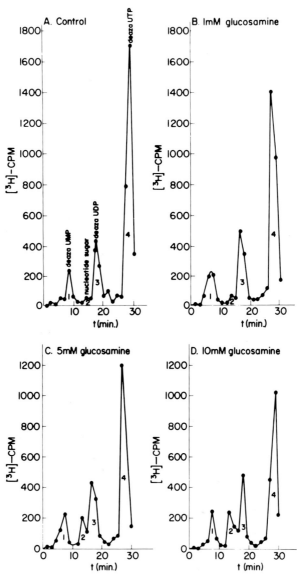

Fig. 7.3 Ribonucleotide pool size analysis of L1210 cells 24 hr after the administration of glucosamine (0, 1, 5, and 10 mM) and 5μCi [³H]-3-deazauridine (DAUR). Peak 1 corresponds to [³H]-deaza-UMP; peak 2 to [³H]-deaza-UDP-sugar; peak 3 to [³H]-deaza-UDP; and peak 4 to [³H]-deaza-UTP. One and five-tenths min fractions were collected from the high-pressure liquid chromatographic column and counted for radioactivity with a Packard TriCarb liquid scintillation counter.

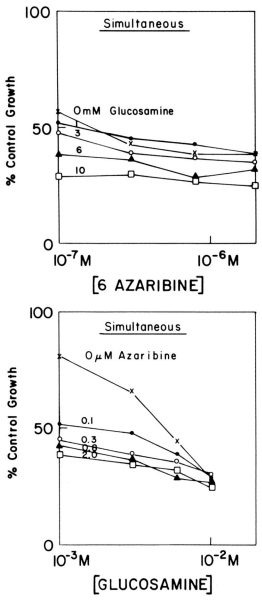

Fig. 7.4 Effects of the simultaneous addition of glucosamine and azaribine on L1210 cell growth after 48 hr. Triplicate cell cultures were set up at each concentration and later counted with a Coulter counter. Data are expressed as the percentage of control growth. Five control cultures were used.

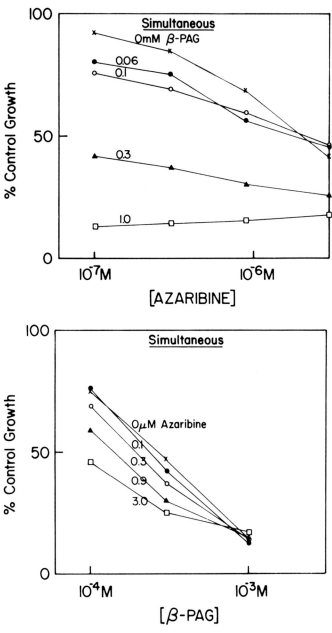

Fig. 7.5 Effects of the simultaneous addition of β-PAG with azaribine on L1210 cell growth. Conditions were similar to those described in the text.

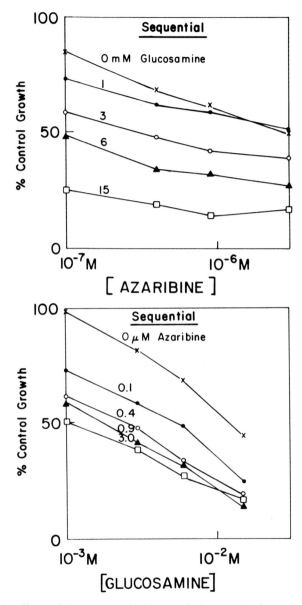

Fig. 7.6 Effects of the sequential addition of glucosamine for 24 hr followed by azaribine for 48 hr. Conditions were similar to those described in the text, with the exception that the glucosamine-containing medium was removed after 24 hr and replaced with medium containing azaribine for 48 hr. Growth was then monitored.

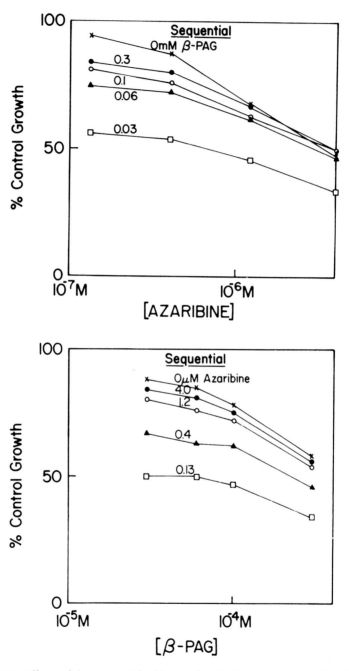

Fig. 7.7 Effects of the sequential addition of β-PAG with azaribine. Conditions were similar to those described in the text.

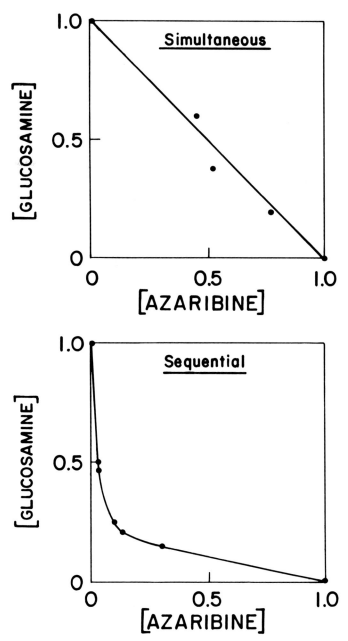

Fig. 7.8 Isobolograms representing the simultaneous and sequential addition of glucosamine with azaribine. Simultaneous addition resulted in additive effects, while sequential addition resulted in a synergistic response.

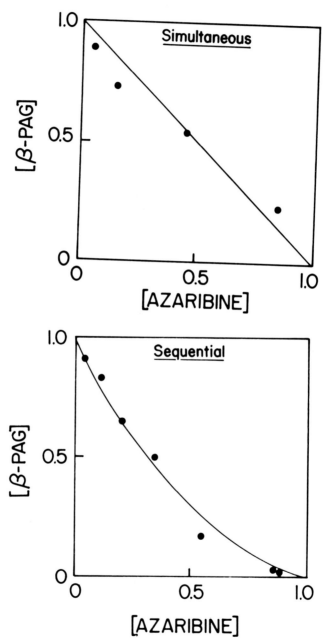

Fig. 7.9 Isobolograms representing the simultaneous and sequential addition of β-PAG with azaribine. Both methods of addition resulted in additive effects.

addition of compounds occurred at time zero, and the cultures were allowed to grow for 48 hr. At that time growth of cultures was monitored using a Coulter counter, and the percentage of control growth was calculated for each combination of agents. A series of growth curves were obtained from which data were obtained to plot the isobologram plots (figs. 7.8 and 7.9). In the sequential studies, various concentrations of glucosamine or β-PAG were added to a series of culture tubes containing L1210 cells and incubated for 24 hr. The glucosamine or β-PAG containing medium was removed and replaced with fresh medium containing various concentrations of azaribine. The cells were then allowed to grow for an additional 48 hr and growth was monitored.

The isobologram plots (fig. 7.8) represent the combination of glucosamine with azaribine. The IC_{50} value for each agent in each study is set to 1.0. Therefore, if it is found that half of the IC_{50} of glucosamine in combination with half of the IC_{50} of azaribine results in a 50% inhibition of control cell growth, a data point is plotted along a straight line joining the two IC_{50} points. This occurred in the case of the simultaneous addition of glucosamine with azaribine, and the effects of this combination were found to be pharmacologically additive. If glucosamine and azaribine were added sequentially, the effects were synergistic, resulting in the concave hyperbolic function also shown in figure 7.8. The addition of β-PAG with azaribine resulted in additive effects, whether the agents were added simultaneously or sequentially (fig. 7.9).

Ribonucleotide pool size analysis was performed on perchloric acid extracts of L1210 cells treated with glucosamine (1 mM), and azaribine (1 μM), either separately or together. Agents were added simultaneously, and the cells were incubated for 3 or 22 hr. At that time the cells were washed and extracted with 6% perchloric acid, as previously described (32, 41). Ribonucleotide pools were determined, and each peak was integrated and compared with control. Results were expressed as the percentage of control (table 7.1).

As can be seen in table 7.1, glucosamine at 1 mM lowered UDP, guanosine diphosphate (GDP), CTP, and UTP pools, while increasing the amount of nucleotide-sugar sixfold within 22 hr. The effects on the uridylate pools were compensated for by increased production of uridine nucleotides. The effects of 1 μM azaribine were more pronounced. All the ribonucleotide pools were lowered with the exception of adenosine 5'-triphosphate (ATP). In fact, the ATP pool was elevated in these cells. On the other hand, the UDP, UDP-sugar, GDP, CTP, and UTP pools were all significantly lowered. The simultaneous addition of glucosamine and azaribine resulted in further decreases in UTP and CTP. The CTP pool fell to 17% of control within 3 hr and to 11% at 22 hr following exposure

Table 7.1 L1210 Ribonucleotide pool sizes following chemotherapy with glucosamine plus azaribine

	Pool Sizes (Percentage of Control)*					
Ribonucleotide	*Glucosamine (1 mM)*		*Azaribine (1 μM)*		*Glucosamine Plus Azaribine (Simultaneous)*	
	3 hr	*22 hr*	*3 hr*	*22 hr*	*3 hr*	*22 hr*
UDP	96	57	70	26	75	27
ADP	104	86	105	89	106	88
UDP-Sugar	134	600	63	67	87	80
GDP	51	60	36	29	32	35
CTP	50	89	50	67	17	11
UTP	69	82	41	61	33	14
ATP	88	114	113	148	116	137
GTP	75	122	69	94	113	86

*Pool sizes were measured using high-pressure liquid chromotography on the acid-soluble fractions from L1210 cells treated with the agents listed in the left column. Areas under each curve were integrated, and each pool was compared as a percentage of control.

to the combination of glucosamine and azaribine. UTP pools fell to 14% of control within 22 hr. These effects on UTP and CTP may explain the additive and synergistic effects observed with the combinations of glucosamine and azaribine. Glucosamine administration results in the formation of large amounts of UDP-sugar, necessitating an increase in the de novo biosynthesis of uridine. Azaribine blocks de novo synthesis of uridine, thereby preventing maintenance of adequate intracellular uridine nucleotide pools. When these agents are added together, the existing pool of UTP is lowered with no compensatory increase in synthesis of uridine. This results in a severe deficiency of uridine nucleotides and a corresponding decrease in the CTP pool, which is dependent on UTP. Chemotherapy based on this principle may be effective in the treatment of some tumors, especially hepatomas, provided that a suitable rescue therapy of sensitive normal tissues, such as liver, is developed (42).

Glycosyl Transferase Inhibitors

Following the conversion of the phosphosugars to nucleotide-sugars, the sugars are attached covalently to suitable acceptors to form the glycoconjugate. In some cases, the sugars are attached to lipid intermediates that later are involved in the transfer of these sugars to protein, en bloc. Such is the case for dolichol, a polyprenol lipid of long carbon chain length $(C_{80}-C_{100})$, which is involved in the transfer of the core portion of the oligosaccharide chain, via an N-glycosidic linkage (fig. 7.1) to protein (25). Retinol (vitamin A) also has been implicated in the glycosylation process (27), and the administration of 13-*cis*-retinoic acid has been found to decrease the incidence of carcinogen-induced oncogenic transformation (43).

Tunicamycin

A number of antibiotics have been found to interfere with lipid-mediated transfer of sugars to protein. They include tunicamycin (44), amphomycin (45), and bacitracin (46). Tunicamycin, an N-acetyl-glucosamine (glcNAc) containing antibiotic from *Streptomyces lysosuperificus*, has been shown to inhibit the transfer of UDP-glcNAc to dolichol phosphate (44), thereby preventing the transfer of any carbohydrate units to asparagine moieties of protein.

We have examined the antitumor properties of this antibiotic against murine leukemia L1210. Tunicamycin (lot #361-26E-117, a gift from Eli Lilly Laboratories) was found to inhibit L1210 cell growth in vitro by 50% at 2.2×10^{-6}M over 48 hr. At 1.0×10^{-6}M, a nongrowth inhibitory concentration at 24 hr, tunicamycin decreased $[^3H]$-mannose incorporation by more than 40%, decreased $[^{14}C]$-glucosamine incorporation by more than 25%, and decreased $[^3H]$-leucine incorporation by only 16%. L1210 ascites cells were pretreated for 24 hr in vitro with tunicamycin and then inoculated I.P. into DBA/2Ha female mice $(1 \times 10^6$ viable L1210 cells per mouse). Pretreatment with 1.0×10^{-6}M resulted in little or no increase in survival, while cells incubated at concentrations above 1.0×10^{-6}M manifested increased survival times, and all mice receiving cells pretreated with 1.0×10^{-5}M tunicamycin were long-term survivors. Upon reinoculation on day 30 with 1.0×10^6 untreated L1210 ascites cells, the animals were found to be completely resistant to subsequent tumor growth. Tunicamycin pretreatment of L1210 cells was found to be more effective in the establishment of resistance to subsequent tumor growth than neuraminidase pretreatment. There is no significant difference in the tumorigenicity of L1210 cells treated with 1×10^{-5}M tunicamycin and control cells inoculated into mice immunosuppressed by whole-body X-irradiation. These preliminary results indicate that tunicamycin may increase the immunogenicity of tumor cells in syngeneic hosts, and that this effect might be related to its inhibition of the synthesis of specific cell surface glycoproteins (35).

Nucleotide and Nucleotide-Sugar Analogs

Nucleotides have been shown to regulate partially the activity of glycosyl transferases. We found that cytidine 5'-monophosphate (CMP) competitively inhibits sialyltransferase activity (25), and several nucleotide and nucleotide-sugar analogs have been shown to inhibit both ecto-sialyltransferase (32) and human serum sialyltransferase (33).

5'-Fluorocytidine monophosphoric acid acted as a competitive inhibitor of human serum sialyltransferase, having a K_i of 70 μM. This was similar to a K_i of 50 μM for CMP. Enzyme inhibition also was observed with ribodialdehyde CMP and to a lesser extent with 5'-(trans-4-N-acetylcyclohexyl) cytidylic acid hydrochloride and its *cis* counterpart, which were synthesized as analogs of CMP-N-acetylneuraminic acid. We have observed that ribodialdehyde CMP, administered I.P. daily for five days (75 mg/kg/day) to mice one day after I.P. inoculation with 10^6 ascites L1210 tumor cells, increased life span significantly (300%), with most animals being cured of all signs of tumor (34).

Endogenous Inhibitors of Glycosyl Transferases (CAGA)

A purified small-molecular-weight glycopeptide has been isolated from the serums or effusions of cancer patients that inhibits the growth of transformed cells in vitro and in vivo (47). This glycopeptide has been found to be an acceptor molecule for galactosyl transferase that acts as a competitive inhibitor in assay systems, using macromolecular acceptors of galactose as substrates for galactosyl transferase. The source of this molecule in cancer patients' serums is assumed to be the tumor, but the physiological reason for its presence is as yet unknown. It may act in the cancer patient to depress host immune defense mechanisms. Its cytotoxic mechanism of action on tumor cells in vitro is also unknown at this time, although it may be interacting with some growth-regulator site on the tumor cell surface.

Conclusion

The cell surface is an important cellular organelle that is responsible for a number of metabolic events. The cell membrane controls transport and contains numerous receptors and recognition sites responsible for growth control and cell-to-cell communication. Following oncogenic transformation, a number of biochemical differences are observed in the composition of cell surface components. These changes could account for the loss of growth control and further enable the tumor cell to metastasize to other anatomical sites.

In view of these findings, the cell surface must be considered a unique site for chemotherapeutic manipulation. In fact, a number of lipophilic antitumor agents have been found to alter membrane properties. Principal among these are the anthracycline antibiotics, the diacridines, the porphyrins, and the polyene antibiotics (48). These agents have been found to affect cellular agglutination caused by plant lectins, and these findings suggest that qualitative differences exist in membrane structures between transformed and untransformed cell lines. These membrane effects may not account for the cytotoxicity of the agents discussed, especially the DNA intercalators, but they may impart changes in cellular behavior or transport which may account for or improve the selectivity of the agents against tumor cells.

Another class of lipophilic agents currently being evaluated, primarily as drug carriers, are the liposomes. Liposomes, or lipid vesicles, are essentially lipid bilayer sacs capable of trapping and transporting agents to various anatomical sites. They also act as drug depots for the sustained release of chemotherapeutic agents, and some success has been obtained with ara-C-containing liposomes in the treatment of mice with L1210 tumors. Work is currently underway in targeting liposomes to specific tumor sites.

Alternatively, cancer chemotherapy may be directed toward the interference or modification of the biosynthesis of cell surface components. We have pursued this avenue of research by testing a number of membrane sugar, nucleotide, and nucleotide-sugar analogs that may alter membrane glycoconjugate formation or structure. Analogs of glucosamine, galactosamine, mannose, fucose, galactose, and sialic acid have been synthesized and tested for their biological activity. Acetylated amino sugars have been found to be more cytotoxic than their natural counterparts, perhaps due to increased lipid permeability. These amino sugars and their analogs are metabolized to form large amounts of nucleotide-sugar, thereby lowering intracellular ribonucleotide pool sizes. Combination chemotherapy with nucleoside analogs may result in improved therapeutic responses, as found with glucosamine and β-PAG in combination with azaribine. This combination of agents administered sequentially to L1210 leukemic cells in vitro resulted in synergistic responses. Chemotherapy of some leukemias and hepatomas may be obtained with such regimens in vivo.

Direct modification of tumor cells with neuraminidase has resulted in cells with enhanced immunogenic potential. Immunotherapy with neuraminidase-treated allogeneic tumor cells in patients with AML resulted in improved chemotherapeutic responses. We have found that L1210 leukemic cells treated with tunicamycin are more capable of immunizing susceptible syngeneic mice to further L1210 tumor challenge than neuraminidase-treated cells. Tunicamycin interferes with glycoconjugate biosynthesis, and further studies are underway in our laboratory to elucidate the mechanism responsible for this increase in cellular immunogenicity.

Based on the experimental examples discussed in this chapter, it is reasonable to postulate that modification of tumor cell membrane structures by directly acting lipophilic agents or antimetabolites such as sugar analogs or antibiotics may provide a new approach that could be exploited in cancer chemotherapy. This approach may result in improved therapeutic responses in patients. These therapeutic advantages may result from alterations in the structural components of the plasma membrane of cancer cells, leading to an altered regulation of target cell metabolic control or to an altered pattern of the "social behavior" of these cells. Alternatively, improved therapeutic responses following the use of membrane-active agents may be due to increased cancer cell immunogenicity or increased susceptibility of these cells to the mechanisms of host defense.

References

1. Weissman, G., and Claiborne, R. *Cell membranes.* New York: HP Publishing, 1975.

2. Nicolson, G. L., and Poste, G. The cancer cell: dynamic aspects and modifications in cell-surface organization. *N. Engl. J. Med.* 295:197–203 and 253–258, 1976.

3. Hynes, R. O. Alteration of cell-surface proteins by viral transformation and by proteolysis. *Proc. Natl. Acad. Sci. USA* 70:3170–3174, 1973.

4. Glick, M. C. Cell surface changes associated with malignancy. In *Fundamental aspects of metastasis*, ed. L. Weiss. Amsterdam: North-Holland Publishing Co., 1976.

5. Poste, G., and Papahadjopoulos, D. Lipid vesicles as carriers for introducing materials into cultured cells: influence of vesicle lipid composition on mechanisms of vesicle incorporation into cells. *Proc. Natl. Acad. Sci. USA* 73:1603–1607, 1976.

6. Gregoriadis, G. Targeting of drugs. *Nature* 265:407–411, 1977.

7. Pagano, R. E., and Weinstein, J. N. Interaction of liposomes with mammalian cells. *Annu. Rev. Biophys. Bioeng.* 7:435–468, 1978.

8. Poste, G., and Papahadjopoulos, D. Drug-containing lipid vesicles render drug-resistant tumorous cells senstitive to actinomycin D. *Nature* 261:699–701, 1976.

9. Juliano, R. L., and Stamp, D. Pharmacokinetics of liposome-encapsulated anti-tumor drugs. *Biochem. Pharmacol.* 27:21–27, 1978.

10. Mayhew, E. et al. Inhibition of tumor cell growth *in vitro* and *in vivo* by 1-β-D-arabinofuranosylcytosine entrapped within phospholipid vesicles. *Cancer Res.* 36:4406–4411, 1976.

11. Weinstein, J. N. et al. Liposomes and local hyperthermia: selective delivery of methotrexate to heated tumors. *Science* 204:188–191, 1979.

12. Murphree, S. A. et al. Effects of adriamycin on surface properties of sarcoma 180 ascites cells. *Biochem. Pharmacol.* 25:1227–1231, 1976.

13. Tritton, T. R.; Murphree, S. A.; and Sartorelli, A. C. Adriamycin: a proposal on the specificity of drug action. *Biochem. Biophys. Res. Commun.* 84:802–808, 1978.

14. Fico, R. M.; Chen, T. K.; and Canellakis, E. S. Bifunctional intercalators: relationship of antitumor activity of diacridines to the cell membrane. *Science* 198:53–56, 1977.

15. Kessel, D. Effects of photoactivated porphyrins at the cell surface of leukemia L1210 cells. *Biochemistry* 16:3443–3449, 1977.

16. Medoff, G. et al. Synergistic effect of amphotericin B and 1, 3-bis (2-chloroethyl)-1-nitrosourea against a transplantable AKR leukemia. *Cancer Res.* 34:974–978, 1974.

17. Bekesi, J. G., St. Arneault, G.; and Holland, J. F. Increase of leukemia L1210 immunogenicity by *Vibrio cholerae* neuraminidase treatment. *Cancer Res.* 31:2130–2132, 1971.

18. Simmons, R. L., and Rios, A. Immunotherapy of cancer: immunospecific rejection of tumors in recipients of neuraminidase treated tumor cells plus BCG. *Science* 174:591–593, 1971.

19. Holland, J. F., and Bekesi, J. G. Immunotherapy of human leukemia with neuraminidase-modified cells. *Med. Clin. North Am.* 60:539–548, 1976.

20. Patterson, M. K., Jr. L-Asparaginase: basic aspects. Pp. 695–722 in *Antineoplastic and immunosuppressive agents*, part II, ed. A. C. Sartorelli and D. G. Johns. Berlin: Springer-Verlag, Berlin, 1975.

21. Bosmann, H. B., and Kessel, D. Inhibition of glycoprotein synthesis in L51784 mouse leukemic cells by L-asparaginase *in vitro. Nature* 226:850–851, 1970.

22. Kessel, D., and Bosmann, H. B. Effects of L-asparaginase on protein and glycoprotein synthesis. *FEBS Lett.* 10:85–88, 1970.

23. Sobin, L. H., and Kidd, J. G. Alterations in protein and nucleic acid metabolism of lymphoma 6C3HED-OG cells in mice given guinea pig serum. *J. Exp. Med.* 123:55–73, 1966.

24. Spiro, R. G., Spiro, M. J.; and Adamany, A. M. Enzymic assembly of the carbohydrate units of glycoproteins and the role of lipid intermediates. *Biochem. Soc. Symp.* 40:37–55, 1974.

25. Bernacki, R. J. Regulation of rat-liver glycoprotein: N-actyneuraminic acid transferase activity by pyrimidine nucleotides. *Eur. J. Biochem.* 58:477–481, 1975.

26. Waechter, C. J., and Lennarz, W. J. The role of polyprenol-linked sugars in glycoprotein synthesis. *Annu. Rev. Biochem.* 45:95–112, 1976.

27. DeLuca, L. M. The direct involvement of vitamin A in glycosyl transfer reactions of mammalian membranes. *Vitam. Horm.* 35:1–57, 1977.

28. Paul, B., and Korytnyk, W. Cell surface as a target for chemotherapy: potential inhibitors of biosynthesis of the protein-carbohydrate linkage in glycoproteins. Pp. 311–336 in *Cell surface carbohydrate chemistry*, ed. R. E. Harmon. New York: Academic Press, Inc., 1978.

29. Sharma, M., and Korytnyk, W. A general and convenient method for synthesis of 6-fluoro-6-deoxyhexoses. *Tetrahedron Letters* 6:573–576, 1977.

30. Sufrin, J. et al. Halogenated L-fucose and D-galactose analogues: synthesis and metabolic effects. *J. Med. Chem.* 23: 143–149, 1980.

31. Bernacki, R. J. et al. Biochemical characteristics, metabolism, and anti-tumor activity of several acetylated hexosamines. *J. Supramol. Struct.* 7:235–250, 1977.

32. Bernacki, R. J. et al. Plasma membrane as a site for chemotherapeutic intervention. Pp. 217–237 in *Advances in enzyme regulation,* ed. G. Weber. Oxford: Pergamon Press, 1978.

33. Klohs, W. D.; Bernacki, R. J.; and Korytnyk, W. Effects of nucleotides and nucleotide: analogs on human serum sialyltransferase. *Cancer Res.* 39:1231–1238, 1979.

34. Korytnyk, W. et al. CMP and CMP-sugar analogs as inhibitors of sialic acid incorporation into glycoconjugates. *Eur. J. Med. Chem.,* 15:77–84, 1980.

35. Morin, M., and Bernacki, R. J. Biochemical and biological effects of tunicamycin on murine L1210 leukemia. *Proc. Am. Assoc. Cancer Res.* 20:192, 1979.

36. Handschumacher, R. E. et al. Summary of current information on 6-azauridine. *Cancer Chemother. Rep.* 21:1–11, 1962.

37. Jackson, R. C.; Williams, J. C; and Weber, G. Enzyme pattern-directed chemotherapy: synergistic interaction of 3-deazauridine with D-galactosamine, *Cancer Treat. Rep.* 60:835–843, 1976.

38. Keppler, D. Uridine triphosphate deficiency, growth inhibition, and death in ascites hepatoma cells induced by a combination of pyrimidine biosynthesis inhibition with uridylate trapping. *Cancer Res.* 37:911–917, 1977.

39. McPartland, R. P. et al. Cytidine 5'-triphosphate synthetase as a target for inhibition by the anti-tumor agent 3-deazauridine. *Cancer Res.* 34:3107–3114, 1974.

40. Rustum, Y. M. et al. Multifactorial cellular determinants of the action of antimetabolites. *Adv. Enzyme Regul.* 14:281–295, 1976.

41. Rustum, Y. High pressure liquid chromatography: 1. Quantitative separation of purine and pyrimidine nucleosides and bases. *Anal. Biochem.* 90:289–299, 1978.

42. Keppler, D. Approaches to the chemotherapy of hepatomas. Pp. 485–492 in *Falk symposium 25,* ed. H. Remmer, H. M. Bolt, P. Bannasch, and H. Popper. MTP Press, 1978.

43. Sporn, M. B. et al. 13-*Cis*-retinoic acid: inhibition of bladder carcinogenesis in the rat. *Science* 195:487–489, 1977.

44. Lehle, L., and Tanner, W. The specific site of tunicamycin inhibition in the formation of dolichol-bound N-acetylglucosamine derivatives. *FEBS Lett.* 71:167–170, 1976.

45. Kang, M. S.; Spencer, J. P.; and Elbein, A. D. Amphomycin inhibits the incorporation of mannose and glcNAc in lipid-linked saccharides by aorta extracts. *Biochem. Biophys. Res. Commun.* 82:568–574, 1978.

46. Spencer, J. P.; Kang, M. S; and Elbein, A. D. Inhibition of lipid-linked

saccharide synthesis by bacitracin. *Arch. Biochem. Biophys.* 190:829–837, 1978.

47. Podolsky, D. K.; Weiser, M. M.; and Isselbacher, K. J. Inhibition of growth of transformed cells and tumors by an endogenous acceptor of galactosyl-transferase. *Proc. Natl. Acad. Sci. USA* 75:4426–4430, 1978.

48. Hatten, M. E., and Burger, M. M. Effect of polyene antibiotics on the lectin-induced agglutination of transformed and untransformed cell lines. *Biochemistry* 18:739–745, 1979.

Chapter 8

Cellular Interactions and the Expression of the Malignant Phenotype

John S. Bertram, Ph.D.

Introduction

Current cancer therapy by drugs or radiation is plagued by a lack of specificity in the proximal target of action in malignant cells. The drugs in use possess toxicity toward both host cells and target cells because the mode of action of most chemotherapeutic agents is to damage DNA or inhibit the synthesis of DNA and/or RNA. Since host cells depend on the integrity of these macromolecules to the same extent as malignant cells, this lack of specificity, or low therapeutic index, is not surprising. In spite of these formidable drawbacks, chemotherapeutic agents are proving relatively effective in certain types of neoplastic diseases, primarily leukemias. Success appears to be in part due to the high proportion of tumor cells undergoing proliferation; to the existence of a stem cell population of host cells, which are not in the proliferative stage of the cell cycle and are thus largely protected from the cytotoxic action of these drugs; and to quantitative differences in the profile of multiple biochemical parameters affecting drug action in different target cells.

Evidence for Cellular Interactions In Vivo

Chemotherapy of solid tumors has had more limited success, and one of the major reasons for poor therapeutic response is probably the existence within the primary tumor or its metastases of a population of nondividing clonogenic cells. The nondividing clonogenic cells behave in many ways like the stem cells of normal tissues such as the bone marrow and intestine, and can be recruited back into the division cycle to repopulate a

105

tumor when the proliferating fraction is destroyed by chemotherapy (1). Successful chemotherapy must exploit some difference in the recruitment time of these tumor "stem" cells vis-à-vis the host stem cells to achieve selectivity of action. The existence of a population of nonproliferating tumor cells runs contrary to the concept that a tumor comprises a mass of cells that do not respond to the physiological biofeedback mechanisms that in normal cells regulate cellular proliferation. The existence of this nonproliferative fraction may most simply be attributed to inadequate vascularization and consequent deprivation of nutrients and accumulation of the products of metabolism. It appears, however, that nonproliferative cell populations do exist in well-vascularized tumors, and these cells are capable of repopulating the primary tumor.

Further evidence that malignant cells may be capable of responding to biofeedback signals comes from the behavior of metastases. These derive from single cells or small clumps of cells which detach from the primary tumor mass, travel in the vascular or lymphatic system, and lodge in a host organ. Many tumors release millions of viable cells into the circulation, but few of these cells survive to produce a metastasis (2, 3). It may take many years for the surviving cells to develop into a clinically demonstrable mass. Metastasis from the breast is perhaps the most vivid example of latent metastasis in which secondary tumors from a primary carcinoma may take many years to become clinically evident. The metastatic tumors that develop possess the same characteristics for progressive growth as the primary tumors removed many years previously. Why have these malignant cells remained dormant for so many years? A striking example of latent metastases comes from the work of Eccles and Alexander (4), in which rats were injected intramuscularly in the leg with a rat sarcoma cell line of known metastatic potential. Amputation of the leg within two weeks of injection resulted in long-term survival rates and no apparent disease. Untreated controls developed lung and lymph node metastases. In the normal course of events, these treated animals would be called tumor-free and cured by the treatment protocol. If these potential long-term survivors were subjected to whole-body irradiation or to drainage of the thoracic duct, however, large numbers of lung and lymph node metastases appeared within a few weeks. This shows that even established highly malignant animal tumor lines can remain latent in vivo for prolonged periods (5). Eccles and Alexander interpreted the mechanism for this latency as being immunological, but clearly other possible explanations exist.

Growth Control Mechanisms

Much of the information on the control of mammalian cell proliferation comes from work with cell cultures of mouse and human fibroblasts.

Unfortunately, in spite of extensive work, the basic mechanisms of cellular growth control in nonmalignant cells are poorly understood. Consequently, aberrations of these controls that must exist in malignant cells are even less well understood.

The basic tool in studies on the growth control mechanism has been cultured fibroblasts, in particular the 3T3 cell lines derived from C3H or Balb/C mice by Todaro and Green (6) and Nilausen and Green (7). These cells and others like them, such as the C3H/10T½CL8 (10T½) line to be described in detail later in this chapter, grow in culture attached to a solid substrate, usually a plastic Petri dish. The cultured fibroblasts are motile and exhibit contact inhibition of movement, which means that cells tend to migrate to areas of low cell density. As long as excess substrate remains, cells divide logarithmically and ultimately completely occupy the surface of the Petri dish. At this point, when cells are surrounded on all sides by other cells and motility is inhibited equally in all directions, cells flatten, cease cell division and form a confluent monolayer of nonproliferating cells. In the 10T½ cell line, this monolayer can be maintained for many months with weekly feeding without any increase in cell number. As seen in figure 8.1, logarithmic cells have a typical fibroblastic morphology with long processes pointing away from the direction of movement. In such a culture, 53% of the cells synthesize DNA during a 1-hr pulse with tritiated thymidine, as demonstrated by autoradiography (8). In contrast, the confluent cells seen in figure 8.2 are well spread on the substrate and form an epithelioid mosaic of cells. In such cultures, less than 2% of the cells undergo DNA synthesis (8). This process can readily be reversed by subculturing cells at low cell densities, which causes the cells to reenter the cell cycle in a parasynchronous wave (9).

In the 10T½ cell line (10) and in selected clones of Balb/3T3 cells (11), neoplastic transformation may be induced in a small proportion of treated cells several weeks after exposure to chemical or physical carcinogens. While the parent line is nontumorigenic under normal circumstances when inoculated into immunosuppressed syngeneic mice, the neoplastic cells produced by carcinogen treatment produce progressively growing sarcomas that eventually kill the host. These neoplastically transformed cells exhibit very different growth characteristics when compared with the cells of origin. The parental cells cease division at confluence and form a stable nonproliferating monolayer, the density of which is determined by the serum concentration in the growth medium, but transformed cells attain much higher saturation densities that are virtually independent of serum concentration (12). These high densities are achieved by the formation of multilayered piles of cells (figs. 8.3 and 8.4). Even when a stable saturation density is achieved by these cells which, as seen in figure 8.5, may be almost tenfold higher than that seen in the nontransformed cells, cell proliferation does not cease (8). Presumably, this high rate of cell

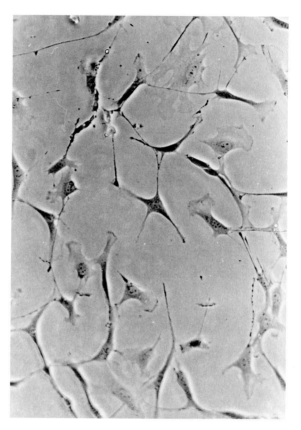

Fig. 8.1 Phase contrast micrograph of logarithmic growth phase 10T½ cells (× 42).

division must be matched by a high rate of cell loss. Transformed cells exhibit a decreased requirement for solid substrates on which to grow; this is manifested by the ability of cells to pile up into multilayered form and to form colonies when suspended in a semisolid medium such as soft agar. There appears to be a high correlation between the ability of a fibroblast to grow in suspension and its ability to form tumors in suitable host animals (13).

The mechanisms by which cells in culture communicate with one another is unclear. Several alternative explanations have been proposed which are beyond the scope of this discussion. It appears to be clear, however, that transformed cells possess several differences in their membranes which may alter the transmission or reception of signals (14) or the use of growth factors (15). Although the actual changes in membrane are not yet fully understood, many researchers in this area have identified

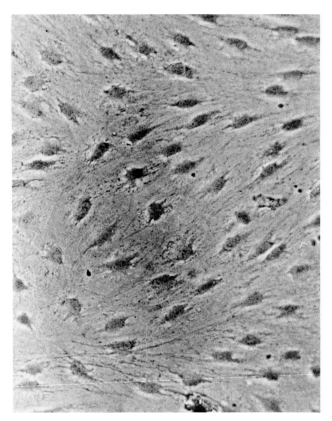

Fig. 8.2 Phase contrast micrograph of confluent 10T½ cells. The regular array of nuclei and the lack of overlapping cell processes is evident (× 29).

deficiencies in tumor cells associated with the synthesis of the saccharide components of membrane proteins and lipids (16). Many researchers using membrane-modified cells in culture and measuring the observed viability of tumor cells have demonstrated that cell membrane oligosaccharides are not required for viability, but act as receptors interacting with hormones and neighboring cells. Such receptors confer blood group antigens (17) and are involved in embryogenesis (18) and probably growth control mechanisms. Loss of these saccharide receptors should thus isolate a cell from its environment and potentially result in unrestrained growth.

This is not to say that the primary lesion that causes transformation is associated with the cell membrane: on the contrary, the stable heritable nature of the transformation and the overwhelming evidence that chemical and physical carcinogens act by causing DNA damage is strong evidence in favor of a primary genetic change. It is through the cell

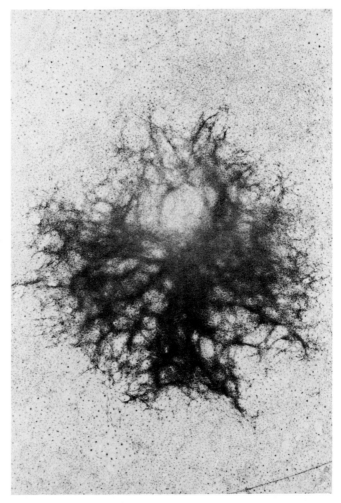

Fig. 8.3 Type III morphologically transformed focus in a culture treated five weeks previously with 3-methylcholanthrene 2.5 μg/ml. The aberrant growth pattern of this focus contrasts strongly with the confluent monolayer of surrounding nontransformed cells. (Methanol fixed and Giemsa stained × 12.)

membrane, however, that a cell interacts with its environment and, if this interaction can be artificially modified, the possibility exists that a genetically transformed cell may be induced to behave normally as long as the modifying stimulus is applied. Several examples of modification demonstrate that, at least in culture, transformed fibroblasts are only conditionally transformed. Many transformed fibroblasts (but not all) are

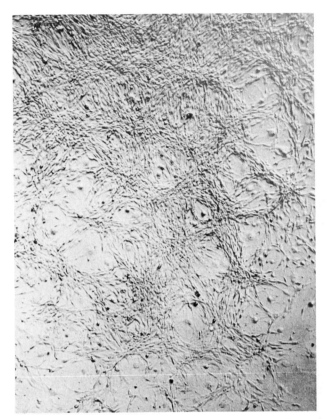

Fig. 8.4 Edge of a type III transformed focus. The transformed cells can be seen to be fairly randomly arranged and to exhibit a high degree of piling up and crossing over of cytoplasmic processes. (Live culture illuminated obliquely × 20.)

deficient in a large molecular weight (220,000) cell-surface glycoprotein known as "fibronectin" (also called "LETS protein," for "large external transformation-sensitive protein"). Studies with fluorescently labeled antibodies to fibronectin have shown that this protein is distributed in an orderly array of fibers over the surface of normal cells and that there is an association of these fibers in the regions of cell-substrate contact. In transformed cells, however, not only is there a decrease in fibronectin, but it is distributed uniformly over the membrane (19, 20). When purified fibronectin is added to cultures of transformed cells (to make up for the deficit), the growth properties of these cells are altered. Cells become more flattened like their normal counterparts, but cell division is not inhibited (21). If, instead of a cell-surface glycoprotein, one adds succinyl-concanavalin A, a chemically modified plant lectin, nontransformed 3T3 cells

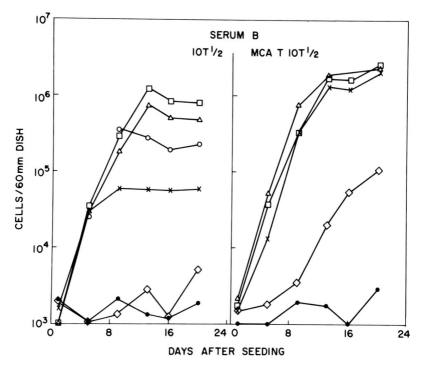

Fig. 8.5 Growth curves for cells cultured in serum. On day 0, 5 × 10³ 10T½ cells (left panel) or 3-methylcholanthrene-transformed cells (right panel) were seeded in 60 mm Petri dishes in Eagle's basal medium (BME) supplemented with the following concentrations of heat-inactivated fetal calf serum Lot A750318: 20%, □; 10%, Δ; 5%, O; 2.5%, X; 1%,◊; and 0.1%, ●. Cultures were refed with the appropriate serum every three to four days. Total cells per dish were determined starting 24 hr after seeding. Results represent the means of four dishes. Reproduced by permission of *Cancer Res.* (12).

reach confluence at lower cell densities corresponding to the amount of lectin added, and transformed cells flatten and cease division at confluence in a manner similar to that of nontransformed cells. These effects are reversible and depend on continued presence of succinyl-concanavalin A (21). Concanavalin A binds to sugars on the cell membrane, specifically gluco- and mannopyranose, at multiple binding sites (22). While the native compound (concanavalin A) is toxic to mammalian cells, chemical modification (succinylation) yields a compound which binds to only two sites and appears to provide a signal on the membrane which masquerades as the signal received by cells when at saturation density. Since transformed cells also become growth-arrested, apparently this signal can be received and acted upon. Neither the nature of this signal nor the subsequent events it triggers are known. Abundant evidence has implicated cyclic nucleotides in this response, however. Nonproliferating cultures of 3T3 cells have higher 3':5'-cyclic adenosine monophosphate (cAMP) levels than either dividing 3T3 cells or virally transformed 3T3 cells (23, 24, 25), while addition of exogenous cAMP has been shown to induce a transient loss of the transformed phenotype in these cells (26, 27). Serum deprivation or growth to high saturation density leads to increased cAMP levels, which decrease rapidly after addition of serum (25) or division to a lower cell density (24) long before an associated increase in DNA synthesis. Conversely, the increase in intracellular cAMP levels by the phosphodiesterase inhibitor theophylline (28), the cyclase stimulator prostaglandin E$_1$ (25), or by addition of exogenous dibutyryl cAMP (29), can cause growth inhibition in normal cells and a temporary inhibition in transformed cells. Cyclic 3':5'-cyclic guanosine monophosphate (uGMP) (30) or levels of the respective phosphodiesterases generally show inverse relationships with growth state.

Cellular Interactions in the C3H/10T½ Cell Line

Researchers whose studies are described in this section used a line of mouse embryo fibroblasts designated C3H/10T½CL8 (10T½), which was developed in Dr. Heidelberger's laboratory (31). This line is highly sensitive to postconfluence inhibition of cell division and becomes growth arrested at low saturation densities (fig. 8.5, left panel). We found that when these cells were exposed to a carcinogenic chemical when in the logarithmic growth phase and then allowed to reach confluence, a small percentage of cells, depending on the concentration of carcinogen employed, became morphologically transformed. The transformants failed to cease division at the saturation density of normal 10T½ cells and formed piled-up foci of fusiform cells (fig. 8.5, right panel). With increasing time in culture, these foci spread over surrounding nontransformed cells and took over the entire culture dish. When such foci were cloned and injected into syngeneic immunosuppressed C3H mice, it was found that sarcomas developed at the injection site. Injection of parental 10T½ cells does not produce sarcomas. Thus, the morphological transformation resulting from carcinogen exposure was demonstrated to be malignant transformation (10). The 10T½ cell line is currently being used in many laboratories in this country and elsewhere.

In studies designed to improve the sensitivity of this assay system as a quantitative test for carcinogenic activity (12), we observed that by reducing the concentration of heat-inactivated fetal calf serum in the growth medium from 10 to 5% (and thereby concomitantly reducing the saturation density of normal cells, see figure 8.5), we allowed the phenotypic expression of transformed cells otherwise held latent by the culture conditions. Conversely, by increasing the concentration of heat-inactivated fetal calf serum to 15%, all cells initiated by a transforming concentration of dimethylbenzanthracene (DMBA) were made latent by the culture conditions. Since cultures were all exposed to the carcinogen under identical conditions of serum concentration, this effect could not be caused by differences in reaction of the carcinogen with the cell, nor could it be due to a selective cytotoxicity of serum to transformed cells, since by switching the serum concentration from high (nonpermissive) to low (permissive), all the hitherto latently transformed cells were able to express their transformed potential (table 8.1). Thus high serum concentration and/or the high cell density induced by high serum concentration was capable of repressing the phenotype of de novo carcinogen-transformed cells.

We next set up reconstruction experiments to determine whether this effect was limited to de novo transformed cells that had never expressed the transformed phenotype or could be extended to malignantly transformed cell lines that exhibited all the criteria of transformation and were tumorigenic in vivo. In these experiments, we seeded 100 malignantly transformed cells onto confluent monolayers of 10T½ cells grown to confluence in various serum concentrations. To rule out any direct cytotoxic effects of serum on the transformed cells, we also plated these cells into Petri dishes containing the various serum concentrations but not containing 10T½ cells. As shown in figure 8.6 (lower panels), in dishes containing confluent 10T½ cells the malignantly transformed cells grew to form large foci when cultured in low (2.5%) serum, but failed to form foci, or formed smaller foci, when cultured in high (20%) serum. That this was not due to a direct effect of serum is shown in the upper panels of figure 8.6, where it can be seen that in the absence of 10T½ cells, transformed cells grew less well in 2.5% serum. To rule out the possibility that transformed cells were in fact producing large foci in mixed cultures but that these were masked by the high concentration of serum, we trypsinized some cultures and suspended the single cells so produced in a semisolid growth medium. Under these conditions the nontransformed cells, which require glass or plastic on which to spread and grow, failed to produce colonies, whereas the transformed cells that had lost this requirement produced colonies suspended in the semisolid growth medium. The results of this study, seen in figure 8.6, show that as the serum concentration increased, the number of cells clonogenic in semisolid medium (transformed cells) decreased. It is of interest that for cell line A (lower left

Table 8.1   Reversibility of the serum-induced inhibition of the transformed phenotype

Treatment	Serum Concentration 8 Days Posttreatment	Final Serum Concentration Days Posttreatment	Transformed Foci/ Dish ± Standard Error
Acetone control	10	10	0
Acetone control	5	5	0
DMBA	5	5	2.0 + 0.31
DMBA	10	10	1.2 + 0.47
DMBA	15	15	0
DMBA	15	5 (22)*	1.9 + 0.41
DMBA	15	5 (29)	1.6 + 0.39

SOURCE: Reproduced with permission of *Cancer Res.* (12).

NOTE: Replicate cultures in Eagle's basal medium (BME) plus 10% serum were treated with dimethylbenzanthracene (DMBA) (0.5 μg/ml) or acetone as a control. After 8 days, groups of 12 cultures were exposed to 5, 10, or 15% serum. Those cultures exposed to 5 and 10% serum were maintained at that level for a further 28 days, then fixed, stained, and scored. Those cultures exposed to 15% serum were either fixed after 28 days or exposed for 28 days to 5% serum at increasing time intervals after treatment.

*Numbers in parentheses are cultures exposed to 5% serum at increasing time intervals after treatment with 15% serum.

panel), cultured in 20% serum, no foci were visible on the confluent monolayer of 10T½ cells, yet a few cells were present which formed colonies in semisolid medium. When replicate cultures were exposed to permissive concentrations of 5% serum, foci again reappeared, demonstrating that these clonogenic cells can express their transformed phenotype and that somehow a state of reversible growth arrest is induced in these cells by normal cells. This effect requires cell-to-cell contact, or at least close proximity, since growth medium removed from nonpermissive cultures is not inhibitory to the growth of transformed cells. On the contrary, cell growth is enhanced (table 8.2).

In an attempt to define the nature of the communication between 10T½ cells and their transformed counterparts, we investigated the role played by cyclic nucleotides in this response (32). Many laboratories have reported that there is a relationship between high cAMP levels and growth arrest of fibroblasts, and that some aspects of the normal phenotype may be induced in transformed fibroblasts by agents that increase cAMP levels.

We found that cAMP itself or dibutyryl cAMP failed to affect the growth of transformed cells in reconstruction experiments set up as described previously. Drugs known to inhibit phosphodiesterase, the enzyme responsible for destroying cAMP, however, were found to produce effects similar to the effects of serum described previously. In both de novo

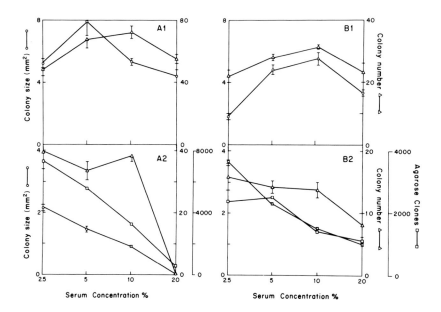

Fig. 8.6 Effect of serum concentration on the growth of transformed cells in the presence and the absence of 10T½ cells. Confluent cultures of 10T½ cells were prepared by seeding 10^4 cells in the stated serum concentrations. When confluent, as judged microscopically, 5 ml of fresh medium supplemented with the appropriate serum concentration were added to the confluent monolayers and to an equal number of empty dishes. All dishes were seeded 24 hr later with transformed cells. Dishes were incubated for about eight days without further medium change. At this time dishes were scored for colony number (Δ) and colony size (O), and in the case of the mixed cultures, the contents of two dishes were seeded into agarose to determine the number of clonogenic cells (□). Clone A (left panels) was a malignantly transformed 3-methylcholanthrene line at passage 72 when used; clone B (right panels) was a recently isolated 3-methylcholanthrene-transformed line. In upper panels (A1, B1), cells were seeded in the absence of 10T½ cells; in lower panels (A2, B2), cells were seeded onto confluent monolayers of 10T½ cells. Results represent the mean ± standard error for colony number and area and the mean of two cultures each for the clonogenicity in agarose.
Reproduced by permission of *Cancer Res.* (12).

Table 8.2 Comparative effects of new medium versus used medium on
the growth and plating efficiency of transformed cells

Cell Line	Medium	Plating Efficiency (Percentage)*	Size ± Standard Error (mm²)*
A	5% new	46 ± 2.5	0.8 ± 0.2
A	5% used	58 ± 12.0	2.0 ± 0.2†
A	20% new	53 ± 4.2	1.0 ± 0.1
A	20% used	50 ± 6.3	1.7 ± 0.1†
B	5% new	51 ± 2.8	2.2 ± 0.2
B	5% used	78 ± 3.5	3.0 ± 0.3†
B	20% new	32 ± 2.1	2.2 ± 0.2
B	20% used	60 ± 4.2	2.1 ± 0.2

SOURCE: Reproduced with permission of *Cancer Res.* (12).

NOTE: Seven-day-old culture medium was aspirated from cultures of 10T½ cells grown to confluency in 20% and in 5% serum and subsequently overlaid with the transformed cell line A or B. At the time of aspiration, the transformed cells had produced large colonies in 5% serum but not in 20% serum. The used medium was centrifuged and poured into empty Petri dishes; identical dishes were prepared using fresh medium containing 5 or 20% serum. Transformed cells were then placed in respective dishes of used medium and corresponding dishes of new medium, and cell growth was measured after six days without medium change.

*Mean ± standard error of four dishes.

†Statistically different from corresponding value in new medium.

transformation experiments, in which transformation was induced by 3-methylcholanthrene, and in reconstruction experiments, the phosphodiesterase inhibitors caffeine, theophylline, and isobutylmethylxanthine (IBX) were found to inhibit the expression of the transformed phenotype. As shown in table 8.3, IBX was the most potent compound tested, being active at a concentration of 10^{-5}M. It is also the most potent inhibitor of phosphodiesterase. Even when treatment with IBX was delayed for 21 days after exposure to the carcinogen, 10^{-3} or 10^{-4}M IBX still caused complete inhibition of transformation expression. Transformation can be detected microscopically at about 26 days postcarcinogen. Although 10^{-3}M IBX reduced the growth rate of both nontransformed and transformed 10T½ cells, at a concentration of 10^{-4}M (which was completely effective in inhibiting transformation), no effects of IBX could be detected on cell survival or growth. Thus, cytotoxicity cannot be responsible for the

Table 8.3 Effects of methylxanthines on 3-methylcholanthrene-induced transformation

Drug	Time of Treatment (Days Postcarcinogen)		
	7	14	21
	Foci/Dish (Percentage of 3-Methylcholanthrene Control)		
Caffeine			
10^{-3}M	0	7.9 ± 2	6.4 ± 1
10^{-4}M	63.0 ± 14	80.0 ± 0	85.2 ± 7
Theophylline			
10^{-3}M	2.6	22.3 ± 2	45.6 ± 8
10^{-4}M	81.0 ± 13	56.2 ± 1	72.3 ± 11.7
IBX*			
10^{-3}M	0	0	0
10^{-4}M	0	0	0
10^{-5}M	71.1 ± 13	74.9 ± 16	68.7 ± 18
10^{-6}M	85.3 ± 12	134.1 ± 22	123.3 ± 21

3-Methylcholanthrene 2.5 μg/ml	100 (1.25 ± 0.4 foci/dish) experiment 1
Control	100 (2.1 ± 0.5 foci/dish) experiment 2

SOURCE: Reproduced with permission of *Cancer Res.* (32).

NOTE: Replicate cultures were treated with 3-methylcholanthrene 2.5 μg/ml for 24 hr 1 day after seeding. Seven, 14, or 21 days after removal of the carcinogen, the appropriate concentration of the appropriate methylxanthine was added and was maintained in the culture for the 36-day duration of the experiment. Results represent the means ± standard error of the mean of two separate experiments, each using 12 dishes/data point. No transformation was observed in acetone- or methylxanthine-treated controls.
*Isobutylmethylxanthine.

observed effects. This conclusion is underlined by the demonstration that the effects of IBX are reversible, as illustrated in figure 8.7. The effects of increasing duration of exposure to 10^{-4} and 10^{-5}M IBX are plotted in figure 8.7. All treatments started seven days after exposure to 3-methylcholanthrene. Continuous exposure to the drug was required to produce the maximum inhibition of transformation, and removal of the drug followed by a sufficient post-treatment expression time allowed latently transformed cells to express their transformed phenotype. As with high serum, cell-to-cell contact is apparently required for the inhibitory effects of IBX, since conditioned medium containing 10^{-4}M IBX removed from

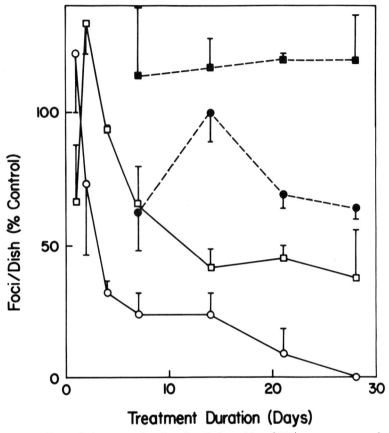

Fig. 8.7 Effect of duration of isobutylmethylxanthine (IBX) treatment on the development of 3-methylcholanthrene-induced transformed foci. Replicate cultures were treated with 3-methylcholanthrene 2.5 μg/ml for 24 hr 1 day after seeding. Seven days after removal of carcinogen, replicate cultures were exposed to IBX 10^{-4}M (O) or 10^{-5}M (□) for periods of 1–28 days, at which point all cultures were fixed and stained. A separate series of cultures were exposed to IBX 10^{-4}M (●) or 10^{-5}M (■) for a period of 7–28 days, and these cultures were fixed and stained 28 days after removal of IBX, to allow expression of latent foci. Results represent the means plus standard error of the mean of three separate experiments, each using 12 dishes/data point. Reproduced with permission of *Cancer Res.* (32).

10T½ cultures was not growth inhibitory for malignant cells. Again, as demonstrated previously using serum concentration as a modulator of cellular interactions, the effects of IBX could also be demonstrated in reconstruction experiments, indicating that both serum and IBX do not simply inhibit the progression of carcinogen-initiated cells to malignancy, but somehow increase the degree of communication between normal and transformed cells in culture.

What form this communication takes is not clear, but intimate cellular contact is required. We have shown that IBX causes profound elevations of cAMP levels in both cells and their growth medium (table 8.4), and that there is a good correlation between concentrations of IBX causing elevations in cAMP and concentrations active in inhibiting expression of transformation (table 8.3). It should be noted, however, that exogenous cAMP or dibutyryl cAMP added to cultures in a manner similar to the addition of IBX were not very effective inhibitors of transformation expression. From this one may conclude either that IBX has effects in addition to effects on cAMP metabolism, or that IBX induces effects on specific compartments of cAMP which cannot be duplicated by exogenously added cAMP.

Mechanisms of Intracellular Communication

It is unclear how intracellular communication between normal and transformed cells occurs. All evidence points to the conclusion that in mixed cultures, transformed cells are growth arrested under permissive conditions. This in itself is remarkable, since in nonmixed cultures transformed cells grow to high cell densities with no proliferation rate restriction (8), and attempts to cause growth inhibtion by depleting the growth medium of serum and isoleucine (8), or of Ca^{++} (33) have shown that transformed 10T½ cells continue to proliferate until highly limiting conditions are reached. These findings suggest that the cocultivated 10T½ cells reestablish some form of physiological growth control in malignant cells. As a working hypothesis, we currently are investigating the role of direct transfer of information molecules between cells. Pathways of low resistance have been demonstrated between touching cells through which electrical impulses, ions and dyes, and small molecules up to about 1,000 daltons in size (34) may diffuse. This form of communication can occur both in vivo and in vitro. There is now persuasive evidence that this transfer occurs via gap junctions, which can be observed under transmission electron microscopy as regions of close approximation of the plasma membranes of adjacent cells. These regions can be seen by freeze fracture techniques as areas of dense intramembranous particles, which on lanthanum staining are revealed as an array of 8-nm pits or pores. Because these junctions act as a network of interconnecting channels, molecules produced by one cell can diffuse widely (35). Communication between malignant cells is much reduced or absent completely, while communication between normal and malignant cells may occur at intermediate levels

Table 8.4 Isobutylmethylxanthine (IBX) concentration (M)

	0	10^{-4}	10^{-5}	10^{-6}
	*pmole cAMP/10^6 Cells**			
Cells				
Experiment 1	0.21 ± 0.02	1.12 ± 0.04†	0.37 ± 0.06†	0.24 ± 0.01
Experiment 2	0.49 ± 0.16	1.80 ± 0.17	0.60 ± 0.08	0.48 ± 0.01
Experiment 3	9.22 ± 0.04	0.70 ± 0.12	ND‡	ND
	pmole cAMP/5 ml Culture Medium			
Medium				
Experiment 1	7.51 ± 1.5	79.7 ± 5.8†	36.6 ± 3.1†	11.2 ± 0.8
Experiment 2	14.81 ± 1.7	107.9 ± 3.5†	24.3 ± 1.7†	12.1 ± 0.05
Experiment 3	3.68 ± 0.8	37.5 ± 9.1†	ND	ND

SOURCE: Reproduced with permission of *Cancer Res.* (32).
NOTE: Elevation of cAMP levels by IBX in 10T½ cells and in their growth medium. Confluent 10T½ cells were treated with the stated concentration of IBX or solvent control for 72 hr, at which time cells and supernatant medium were assayed for cAMP by radioimmunoassay as described in the text. Results represent the mean ± standard error of the mean of four measurements, each made on three replicate cultures.
*cAMP = 3':5'-cyclic adenosine monophosphate.
†Significantly different ($p < 0.05$) from respective solvent-only treated controls.
‡ND = not determined.

(36). Mouse L cells, a line of sarcoma-producing transformed fibroblasts, are completely deficient in gap junctions (37), and it is of interest that these cells are not inhibited when cocultivated with 10T½ cells under nonpermissive conditions.

Bell (38) has put forward a theoretical model to explain how tumor cells break through physiological growth control mechanisms and achieve unlimited growth potential. This model assumes the production by normal cells of negative feedback regulators that govern proliferation rate. If the tumor cell responds to but does not secrete this inhibitor, by mathematical modeling Bell was able to demonstrate that a minimum clone size containing 10^3–10^6 cells would be required before cells at the center of this clone would be protected from the locally high levels of inhibitor secreted by adjacent normal cells. Similar conclusions regarding minimum clone size have been reached in studies using the 10T½ cell line. In these studies it was found that expression of transformation could not occur until a transformed focus contained 32–256 cells before contact was made with nontransformed foci (39). While this figure is smaller than that described by Bell, it should be remembered that the in vitro assay is two-dimensional only. Thus the analysis by Bell and by Haber and coworkers (39) supports the concept of a locally diffusable inhibitor, and our studies suggest that this inhibitor may be diffusing across membranes, rather than in the extracellular space. It may be supposed that this type of diffusion would allow greater specificity and control, thus permitting an organ or tissue to more closely regulate its architecture.

The significance of the studies discussed here to the clinical situation hinges for the moment on the demonstration that similar communication between normal and malignant cells occur in vivo. As discussed in the introduction to this chapter, there is circumstantial evidence that such communication could be the cause of the prolonged latent period for chemically induced tumors and for the phenomenon of latent metastasis. Experimental studies to investigate such interactions in laboratory animals are currently under way[1]. Should interactions be demonstrated, the way will be open to exploit these modulators of tumor growth. For instance, it may be beneficial to enhance these interactions to delay the development of metastasis until such time as the patient can receive intensive chemotherapy. At this time the interactions could be inhibited in order to stimulate cells rapidly into the cell cycle, where they would be susceptible to cell cycle phase specific agents. At present, these manipulations are only possible in vitro.

References

1. Mendelsohn, M. L. Radiation effects on tumors. In *Radiation research*, ed. G. Gilini. Amsterdam: North-Holland Publishing Co., 1967.

2. Malmgren, R. A. Studies of circulating tumor cells in cancer patients. Pp. 108–117 in *Mechanisms of invasion of cancer*, ed. P. Denoix. New York: Springer-Verlag New York Inc., 1967.

3. Salsbury, A. J. The significance of the circulating cells. *Cancer Treat. Rev.* 2:55–72, 1975.

4. Eccles, S. A., and Alexander, P. Immunologically-mediated restraint of latent tumor metastases. *Nature* 257:52–53, 1975.

5. Wheelock, E. F. et al. The tumor dormant state. Pp. 105–116 in *Progress in cancer research and therapy*, vol. 5, ed. S. B. Day. New York: Raven Press, 1977.

6. Todaro, G. J., and Green, H. Quantitative studies of the growth of mouse embryo cells in culture and their development into established lines. *J. Cell Biol.* 17:299–313, 1963.

---

[1]We have recently determined that IBX administered twice daily to C57B1 mice causes an approximate 10-fold decrease in lung metastases arising from subcutaneously growing or intravenously injected Lewis lung carcinoma cells, and that this therapy is free of major toxicity to the host (40). Supported by USPHS Grant CA 21359.

7. Nilausen, K., and Green, H. Reversible arrest of growth in G_1 of an established fibroblast line (3T3). *Exp. Cell Res.* 40:166–168, 1965.

8. Bertram, J. S.; Libby, P. R.; and LeStourgeon, W. M. Changes in nuclear actin levels with change in growth state of C3H/10T½ cells and the lack of a response in malignantly transformed cells. *Cancer Res.* 37:4104–4111, 1977.

9. Bertram, J. S., and Heidelberger, C. Cell cycle dependency of oncogenic transformation induced by N-methyl-N'nitro-N-nitrosoguanidine in culture. *Cancer Res.* 34:526–537, 1974.

10. Reznikoff, C. A. et al. Quantitative and qualitative studies of chemical transformation of clone C3H mouse embryo cells sensitive to post-confluence inhibition of cell division. *Cancer Res.* 33:3239–3249, 1973.

11. Kakunaga, T. Quantitative system for assay of malignant transformation by chemical carcinogens using a clone derived from Balb/3T3. *Int. J. Cancer.* 12:463–473, 1973.

12. Bertram, J. S. Effects of serum concentrations on the expression of carcinogen-induced transformation in the C3H/10T½CL8 cell line. *Cancer Res.* 37:514–523, 1973.

13. Shin, S. et al. Tumorigenicity of virus transformed cells in nude mice is correlated specifically with anchorage independent growth in vitro. *Proc. Natl. Acad. Sci. USA* 72:4435–4439, 1975.

14. Emmelot, P. Biochemical properties of normal and neoplastic cell surfaces: a review. *Eur. J. Cancer* 9:319–333, 1973.

15. Holley, R. W. A unifying hypothesis concerning the nature of malignant growth. *Proc. Natl. Acad. Sci. USA* 69:2840–2841, 1972.

16. Warren, L.; Bock, C. A.; and Tuszynski, G. P. Glycopeptide changes and malignant transformation: a possible role for carbohydrate in malignant behavior. *Biochim. Biophys. Acta* 516:97–127, 1978.

17. Watkins, W. M. Pp. 830–891 in *Lack of proteins,* 2d ed., ed. A. Gottschalk. Amsterdam: Elsevier-Scientific Publishing Co., 1972.

18. Roseman, S. Sugars of the cell membrane. Pp. 55–64 in *Cell membranes: Biochemistry, cell biology and pathology.* New York: H. P. Publishing Co., Inc., 1975.

19. Mautner, V., and Hynes, R. O. Surface distribution of LETS protein in relation to the cytoskeleton of normal and transformed cells. *J. Cell Biol.* 75:743–768, 1977.

20. Yamada, K. M., and Kennedy, D. W. Fibroblast cellular and plasma fibronectins are similar but not identical. *J. Cell Biol.* 80:492–498, 1979.

21. Mannino, R. J., and Burger, M. M. Growth inhibition of animal cells by succinylated concanavalin A. *Nature* 256:19–22, 1975.

22. Poretz, R. D., and Goldstein, I. J. An examination of the topography of the saccharide binding sites of concanavalin A and of the forces involved in complexation. *Biochemistry* 9:2890–2896, 1970.

23. Granner, D. et al. Tyrosine aminotransferase: enzyme induction independent of adenosine 3',5'-monophosphate, *Science* 162:1018–1020, 1968.

24. Sheppard, J. R. Differences in the cyclic adenosine 3', 5'-monophosphate levels in normal and transformed cells. *Nature N. B.* 236:14–16, 1972.

25. Otten, J.; Johnson, G. S.; and Pastan, I. Cyclic AMP levels in fibroblasts: relationship to growth rate and contact inhibition of growth. *Biochem. Biophys. Res. Commun.* 44:1192–1198, 1971.

26. Sheppard, J. R. Restoration of contact inhibited growth to transformed cells by dibutyryl adenosine 3', 5'-cyclic monophosphate. *Proc. Natl. Acad. Sci. USA* 68:1316–1320, 1971.

27. Kram, R.; Mamont, P.; and Tomkins, G. M. Pleiotypic control by adenosine 3',5'-cyclic monophosphate: a model for growth control in animal cells. *Proc. Natl. Acad. Sci. USA* 70:1432–1436, 1973.

28. Burk, R. R. Reduced adenyl cyclase activity in a polyoma virus transformed cell line. *Nature* 219:1271–1275, 1968.

29. Johnson, G. S.; Friedman, R. M.; and Pastan, I. Restoration of several morphological characteristics of normal fibroblasts and sarcoma cells treated with adenosine 3',5'-cyclic monophosphate and its derivatives. *Proc. Natl. Acad. Sci. USA* 68:425–429, 1971.

30. Rudland, P. S.; Seeley, M.; and Siefert, W. Cyclic GMP and cyclic AMP levels in normal and transformed fibroblasts. *Nature* 251:417–419, 1974.

31. Reznikoff, C. A.; Brankow, D. W.; and Heidelberger, C. Establishment and characterization of a cloned line of C3H mouse embryo cells sensitive to post-confluence inhibition of cell division. *Cancer Res.* 33:3231–3238, 1973.

32. Bertram, J. S. Modulation of cellular interactions between C3H/10T½CL8 cells and their transformed counterparts by phosphodiesterase inhibitors. *Cancer Res.* 39:3502–3508, 1979.

33. Boynton, A. L. et al. Different extracellular calcium requirements for proliferation of non-neoplastic, preneoplastic and neoplastic mouse cells. *Cancer Res.* 37:2657–2661, 1977.

34. Loewenstein, W. R. Cellular communication by permeable membrane junctions. Pp. 105–114 in *Cell membranes: biochemistry, cell biology and pathology*, ed. G. Weissmann. New York: H. P. Publishing Co., 1975.

35. Revel, J. P., and Karnovsky, M. J. Hexagonal array of subunits in intercellular junctions of the mouse heart and liver. *J. Cell Biol.* 33:C7–C12, 1967.

36. Azarnia, R.; Larsen, W. J.; and Loewenstein, W. R. The membrane junctions in communicating and noncommunicating cells, their hybrids and segregants. *Proc. Natl. Acad. Sci. USA* 71:880–884, 1974.

37. Gilula, N.; Reeves, R.; and Steinbach, A. Metabolic coupling, ionic coupling and cell contacts. *Nature* 235:262–265, 1972.

38. Bell, G. I. Models of carcinogenesis as an escape from mitotic inhibitors. *Science* 192:569–572, 1976.

39. Haber, D. A. et al. Cell density dependence of focus formation in the C3H/10T½ transformation assay. *Cancer Res.* 37:1644–1648, 1977.

40. Janik, P.; Assaf, A.; and Bertram, J. S. Inhibition of growth of primary and metastatic Lewis lung carcinoma cells by the phosphodiesterase inhibitor isobutylmethylxanthine. *Cancer Res.* 40:1950–1954, 1980.

Chapter 9

Ultrastructural Lesions Produced by Anticancer Agents

Carl W. Porter, Ph.D.
Fredika Mikles-Robertson, Ph.D.
and Debora Kramer

Introduction

It is unfortunate that many of the clinically useful anticancer agents must be administered without benefit of knowledge regarding their precise mode of action. Such information would be especially valuable in maximizing the potential of these agents through scheduling, combination chemotherapy, or prevention of adverse side-effects. Ultrastructural studies of cells or tissues treated with a specific anticancer agent can be advantageous as an initial step toward determining the mode of action of the drug. Subtle changes in the morphology of a particular organelle or region of a cell may provide unexpected insight into the intracellular target of the drug and thereby serve to guide subsequent biochemical studies. An ultrastructural lesion resulting from drug treatment is likely to occur earlier than changes in other parameters such as growth inhibition or cell viability, and should therefore be more closely related to primary events caused by the drug. Accordingly, a specific drug-induced lesion may be used to define an early end point for treatment of cells in preparation for biochemical studies.

Unfortunately, the lesions produced by most drugs are either not sufficiently unique or do not occur early enough during treatment to be distinguished from ultrastructural changes associated with general cell death, for example, pyknosis of nuclei or swelling of the endoplasmic reticulum. Yet several anticancer agents have been found to produce unique, distinguishable, ultrastructural lesions that are either consistent with their known mode of action or have led to recognition of additional drug actions.

The antitumor antibiotic adriamycin, for example, introduces a distinct nucleolar lesion that is consistent with the known ability of the drug to inhibit RNA synthesis (1). The effect (fig. 9.1) is similar to that produced by actinomycin D (2) in that it primarily involves the nucleolus. But while actinomycin D and several carcinogens (3) cause a segregation of nucleolar components, adriamycin eventually causes the nucleolus to fragment and disperse throughout the nucleus in much the same manner as lesions induced by the methionine analog, ethionine (4, 5). The effect is attributable to interference with the DNA-RNA template system, since similar nucleolar changes have been induced with ribonuclease (6).

In this chapter an attempt will be made to demonstrate that a number of cancer chemotherapeutic agents produce selective cytological lesions, provided that cell treatment is suitably chosen in order to disassociate specific target effects from general cytotoxicity involving the whole cell. Particular attention will be given to the anticancer agent, methylglyoxal-bis(guanylhydrazone) (MGBG), and how the lesion induced by this agent has been used to clarify our understanding of the mode of action of the

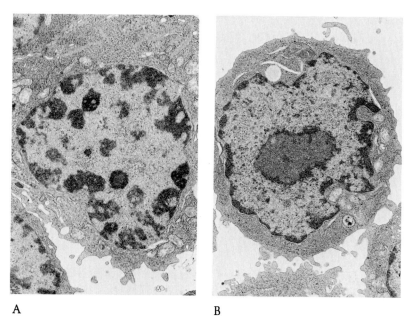

A   B

Fig. 9.1 Electron micrographs of adriamycin-treated (A) and untreated (B) L1210 cells. Note that in the treated cell, the nucleolus is fragmented and dispersed throughout the nucleus, while in the control cell, the nucleolus appears as a consolidated mass in the center of the nucleus. Cells were treated for ½ hr with 50 μg/ml of adriamycin (× 6,000).

drug and of the structurally related molecules, namely the polyamines (fig. 9.2).

Drug Treatment In Vitro

The effects of various anticancer agents on ultrastructure and growth characteristics have been examined in a number of cell lines, including L1210 and P288 murine lymphocytic leukemias, L cell murine fibroblasts, human NALM-1 chronic myelocytic leukemia blast crisis cells (7), and C3H/10T½ mouse embryo fibroblasts (8). By far the most commonly studied cells are the L1210 leukemia cells, which are particularly well suited for ultrastructural studies. The cells grow in suspension culture and do not have to be removed from a substrate; they have a short doubling time (about 12 hr); they display remarkable ultrastructural homogeneity; and individual cells are simple in their ultrastructure yet contain a full complement of easily discernable organelles (i.e., Golgi, mitochrondria, lysosomes, microtubules, vacuoles, endoplasmic reticulum, and nuclear substructures) (fig. 9.3).

In general, murine L1210 leukemia cells are maintained in logarithmic growth as a suspension culture in RPMI 1640 medium containing 10% heat-inactivated dialyzed fetal calf serum with penicillin (100 units/ml) and streptomycin (100 μg/ml). These latter antibiotics do not have an effect on cell ultrastructure at the concentrations employed. Cells are grown in a humidified 5% CO_2 atmosphere at 37°C.

Drug treatment of cells is always initiated while the cells are in logarithmic growth (10^4–10^5 cells/ml). At various times after initiation of drug treatment, cells are removed from flasks for cell density and viability determinations. Cell number is determined by electronic particle counting using a model ZF Coulter counter and is confirmed periodically with hemocytometer estimates. Cell viability is determined by trypan blue dye exclusion (0.5% in saline). Growth kinetic curves are plotted as the number of viable cells against time.

Initial inquiries into the possible effects an anticancer drug might have on cell ultrastructure are routinely conducted at drug concentrations that produce significant (30–100%) growth inhibition but at time points when cell viability as assessed by trypan blue are greater than 80%. This practice ensures that ultrastructural lesions observed with drug treatment are likely to be caused by the drug and not a nonspecific ultrastructural change associated with cell death.

Drug Treatment In Vivo

Murine leukemia L1210 cells are grown in the peritoneums of host DBA/2J mice. An initial inoculum of 10^6 cells in 0.2 cc sterile RPMI 1640

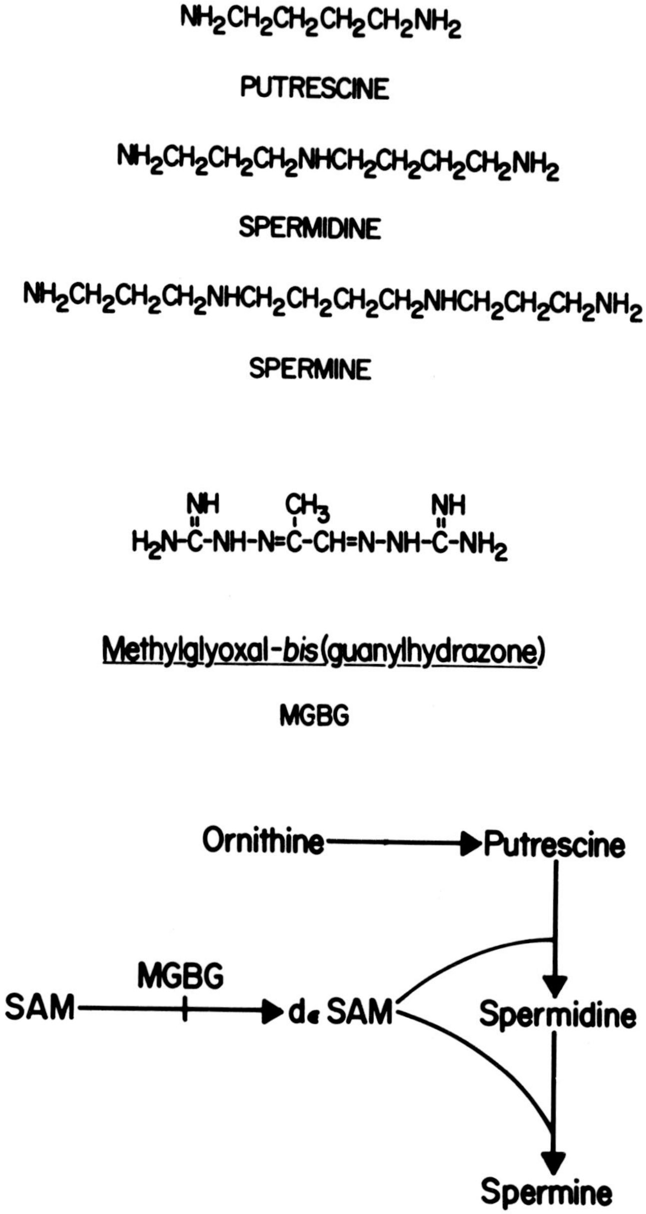

$$NH_2CH_2CH_2CH_2CH_2NH_2$$

PUTRESCINE

$$NH_2CH_2CH_2CH_2NHCH_2CH_2CH_2CH_2NH_2$$

SPERMIDINE

$$NH_2CH_2CH_2CH_2NHCH_2CH_2CH_2CH_2NHCH_2CH_2CH_2NH_2$$

SPERMINE

$$\overset{NH}{\overset{\|}{H_2N-C}}-NH-N=\overset{CH_3}{\overset{|}{C}}-CH=N-NH-\overset{NH}{\overset{\|}{C}}-NH_2$$

Methylglyoxal-*bis*(guanylhydrazone)

A　　　　　　**MGBG**

B

Fig. 9.2 (A) Structural representation of the three most common polyamines and the drug, methylglyoxal-bis(guanylhydrazone) (MGBG). (B) Biosynthetic scheme for polyamines showing the site of action of MGBG at S-adenosylmethionine decarboxylase (SAM).

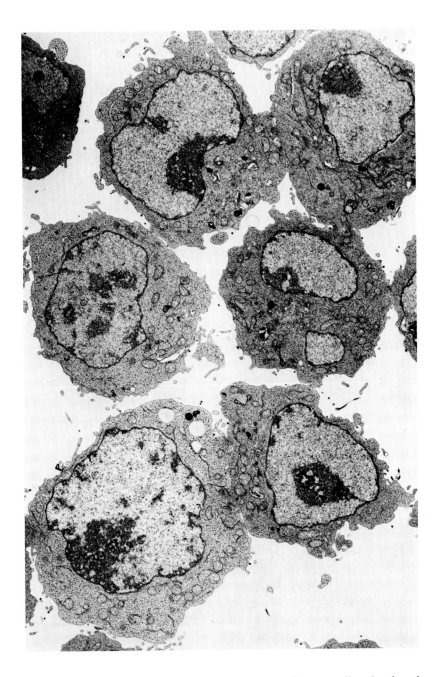

Fig. 9.3 The mitochondria of these control L1210 cells are small, ordered, and have an electron density similar to that of the cytoplasm (× 6,000)

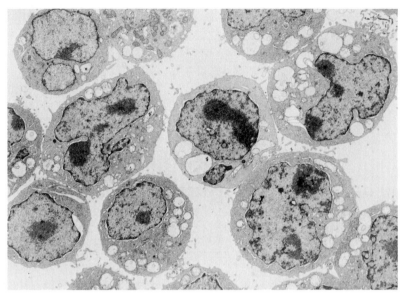

Fig. 9.4 In L1210 cells treated 24 hr with 10 μM MGBG, the mitochondria are characteristically swollen, without cristae, and electron-lucent. All the mitochondria of each cell are affected, and the mitochondrial damage is progressive (× 3,900).

is injected I.P. into each mouse. On day three of cell growth, the mice are injected with the drug. Twenty-four to 48 hr later, the cells are harvested from the ascites fluid, washed twice, and processed for electron microscopy.

Electron Microscopy

Treated and control cell samples (about 10^7 cells) are removed from cultures, washed with cold RPMI 1640, and suspended for 2 hr at 4°C in 3% glutaraldehyde in 0.1 M. phosphate buffer, pH 7.4. Cell pellets are formed by centrifugation and fixed an additional 2 hr. The fixed pellets are washed overnight in phosphate buffer, postfixed in 1% phosphate-buffered osmium tetroxide for 3–4 hr at 4°C, dehydrated in a graded alcohol series, and embedded in Epon-araldite plastic resin. Semithin sections (500 nm) are prepared on a Porter-Blum MT-1 ultramicrotome and stained with 1% toluidine blue O in aqueous sodium borate. Thin sections (about 90 nm) are stained with uranyl acetate/lead citrate and examined with a Siemens Elmiskop 101.

Findings

The ultrastructural effects of a number of anticancer drugs have been examined, but those of the bis(guanylhydrazones) have been especially

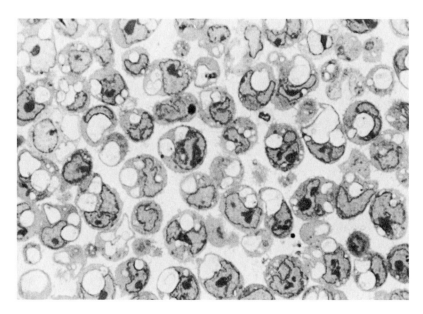

Fig. 9.5 A light micrograph of L1210 cells treated with 10 μM MGBG shows the extent of the damage after 48 hr and the uniformity of the effect among the cell population ($\times$ 1,200).

illustrative for determining the mode of drug action. The bis(guanyl-hydrazones) are a group of compounds in which common terminal amidine groups are separated by variable aliphatic or aromatic structures frequently containing interposed nitrogen groups. Although a number of these compounds are known to possess significant antitumor activity in various experimental systems (9), only the aliphatic derivative MGBG (fig. 9.2A) has attained clinical usefulness in the treatment of human malignancies, acute myelocytic leukemia (AML) in particular (10).

There has been a renewed interest in the clinical potential of MGBG since it was found by the Southwest Oncology Group to be effective against a number of solid tumors that are ordinarily refractory to chemotherapy (11). Although the antiproliferative properties of MGBG have been recognized for many years (9), the mechanism by which the drug effects this action has eluded investigators. Unlike aromatic bis-(guanylhydrazones), which seem to act by binding nuclear DNA, MGBG binds only weakly to DNA and has little effect on DNA polymerase (12). It was discovered recently that the drug causes a profound disturbance in polyamine biosynthesis by inhibiting putrescine-activated S-adenosyl-methionine decarboxylase, a key enzyme in the synthesis of spermidine and spermine (fig. 9.2B) (13, 14). Inhibition of the enzyme in intact cells treated with MGBG causes a rapid increase in intracellular putrescine and a gradual decline in spermidine and spermine pools (fig. 9.2B). Thus far, however, attempts to definitively correlate this effect with the anti-

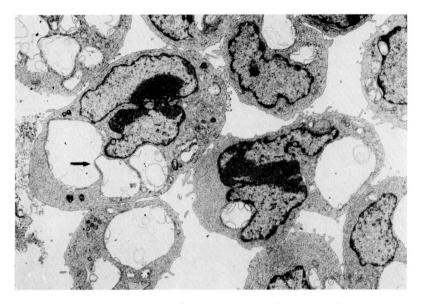

Fig. 9.6 An electron micrograph of the same L1210 cells shown in figure 9.5 show that the vacuoles are, in fact, enormously swollen mitochondria that appear to fuse (arrow) with one another. Even after this treatment, other cellular organelles appear the same as those in the control cells (fig. 9.3) (× 4,900).

proliferative action of MGBG have provided suggestive but inconclusive results (12, 15, 16, 17).

The Effects of MGBG on Cell Ultrastructure

The studies to be described herein were originally prompted by two reports (18, 19) describing the effects of MGBG and polyamines on the ultrastructure of nuclei. Treatment of isolated hepatocyte nuclei with relatively high concentrations (4–10 mM) of MGBG or polyamines resulted in a dispersion of the chromatin and subtle alterations in nucleolar structure. The findings raised the possibility that similar changes would occur in intact cells treated with the drug and could serve as an end point for additional biochemical studies.

Mouse leukemia L1210 cells were treated in culture with growth-inhibitory doses (1–10 μM) of MGBG for 6–48 hr and were examined for ultrastructural damage (20). At the light microscope level, the treatment had little or no effect on nuclear structure but instead gave rise to numerous cytoplasmic vacuoles that occurred uniformly throughout the cell population (fig. 9.5). When examined ultrastructurally, the vacuoles were found to correspond with grossly distended mitochondria (fig. 9.4).

The mitochondria of cells treated with concentrations of MGBG greater than 1.0 μM for longer than 8–12 hr were swollen 4–5 times the size of those in control cell sections (fig. 9.3). The cristae were disorganized and appeared short and inconspicuous. The mitochondrial matrix was electron-lucent and on occasion contained small flocculent densities. It is interesting that the effect seemed progressive with time. That is, the mitochondria continued to enlarge and apparently fuse, so that by 48 hr they occupied up to ⅓ of the cell cytoplasm. Instead of having many small vacuoles, the typical treated cell profile had 1–3 large vacuoles (figs. 9.5 and 9.6). Other cellular organelles, including the nuclear substructure and the microvilli, appeared identical to control cells (fig. 9.3).

Cell viability remained at greater than 85% even at drug doses in which all of the mitochondria in all of the cells appeared to be affected. The first ultrastructurally apparent mitochondrial damage also preceded detectable inhibition of cell growth by several hours, leaving open the possibility of a cause and effect relationship between the two events.

The mitochondrial damage elicited by MGBG was unexpected, although an earlier biochemical study (21) reported an effect of the drug on mitochondrial phosphorylation. These findings raise the possibilities that the mitochondrial damage may be related to the antiproliferative action of the drug or that the mitochondrial damage may be secondary to drug interference with intracellular polyamine pools, in particular spermidine and putrescine. Conceivably, these molecules may be critical to normal mitochondrial function, perhaps at the level of mitochondrial DNA transcription or replication.

Generality of Mitochondrial Damage Among Cultured Cell Types

In order to establish that the mitochondrial damage seen in L1210 cells treated with MGBG was not unique to that particular cell line but was instead a general phenomena among most cultured cell types, the effect of the drug was tested on a variety of cell lines including P288 murine leukemia, L cell fibroblasts, C3H/10T½ mouse embryo fibroblasts (8), and NALM-1 human chronic myelocytic leukemia cells (7). The same ultrastructural lesion occurred in all cases. Mitochondria were swollen, their cristae disorganized, and the matrix became electron-lucent. The drug effect in the NALM-1 cells was peculiar in that, in addition to these changes, the mitochondria developed large electron-dense granules in the matrix (fig. 9.7). Smaller, less conspicuous granules are frequently present in the matrix of normal mitochondria and are generally regarded as depots of certain cations such as calcium (22). While the composition of these structures was not examined in the study just described, it is of interest to

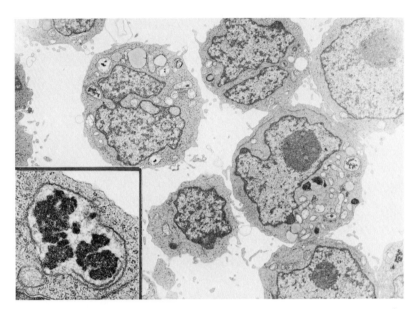

Fig. 9.7 Human NALM-1 cells treated 72 hr with 10 μM MGBG. Note that many of the swollen mitochondria contain electron-dense bodies that, at higher magnification (inset), appear as an amorphous globular substance (× 4,500; inset × 11,500).

note that similar structures also form in the mitochondria of cells treated with relatively high concentrations of the drug ethidium bromide (EB) (fig. 9.8) (23). Other investigators have determined by electron microscope autoradiography and energy-dispersive X-ray microanalysis that these structures contained a complex of EB and mitochondrial DNA (24).

Overall it was concluded that, excepting the granule formation in NALM-1 cells, the effect of MGBG on mitochrondria is the same in cultured human or murine cells and is not peculiar to murine or L1210 cultured cells.

Specificity of the MGBG-Induced Mitochondrial Lesion

The sensitivity of mitochondrial structural change in response to cellular injury caused by a variety of factors is well recognized (25, 26). In such cases, however, it is usual for other cellular organelles, including the cell itself, to swell in response to the injury but not to the same extent as mitochondria. Thus despite the apparent selectivity of MGBG for mitochondria, the possibility was considered that other drugs having a

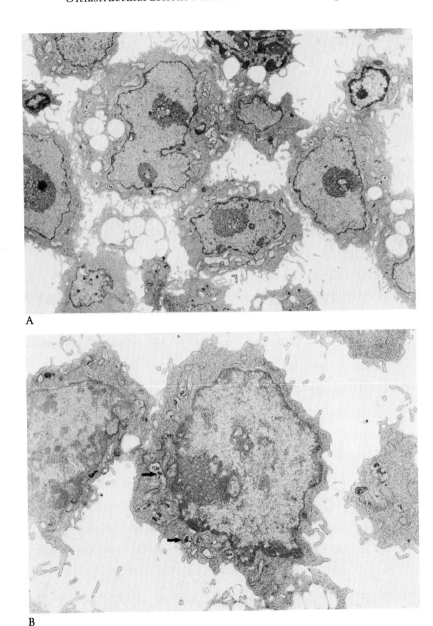

Fig. 9.8 Ascites L1210 cells treated 24 hr in vivo with a single I.P. injection of EB (75 mg/kg). The mitochondria are moderately swollen (A, B) and several contain an electron-dense structure (B arrows). The large clear vacuoles in the cells in A represent lipid vacuoles that are characteristic of ascites but not of cultured L1210 cells (A × 4,000; B × 5,500).

mechanism of action unrelated to that of MGBG might also produce mitochondrial swelling at growth-inhibitory concentrations.

To test this possibility, CCRF-CEM cells, a continuous culture of human lymphoblasts derived from an acute leukemia patient (27), were treated with MGBG or methotrexate and examined ultrastructurally. Methotrexate acts by competitively inhibiting dihydrofolate reductase, thus restricting the availability of tetrahydrofolate to cells for use in single carbon transfer reactions, especially those involved in DNA synthesis (28, 29). The enzyme is cytosolic, therefore its inhibition should not lead to mitochondrial changes unless they are a normal consequence of cell death.

The cells were treated with drug concentrations that gave similar growth inhibition, 10 μM for MGBG and 0.1 μM for methotrexate. Cells treated with MGBG for 24 hr contained mitochondria that were damaged as previously described for other cell types. The mitochondria in the cells treated with metotrexate for up to 72 hr appeared the same as those in control cells and did not appear to be affected by the drug (fig. 9.5). Thus the MGBG reaction in mitochondria appeared to be drug-specific and not due to general drug-induced cell death.

While there was no evidence of mitochondrial damage, the nuclear membrane in cells treated with methotrexate was markedly invaginated, giving rise to numerous infoldings and a highly convoluted cerebriform nucleus (fig. 9.9). The treated cells resembled the characteristic Sézary cells of mycosis fungoides, which appear as mononuclear cells with hyperchromatic folded and indented nuclei (30). Similar structures have also been observed in epithelial cell lines derived from human carcinomas and are regarded, in those cases, as one of several structural parameters for malignancy (31). Lymphocytes from patients with infectious mononucleosis or those stimulated by phytohemagglutinin (PHA) have also been reported to show such nuclear changes (32), but they are not nearly so dramatic as those seen with methotrexate treatment or in Sézary cells (30). The nuclear changes were unexpected, especially since in previous studies ultrastructural changes in liver exposed to methotrexate were confined mainly to cytoplasmic organelles, and no nuclear alterations were noted (33, 34). Interestingly, nuclear changes were not seen in murine leukemia L1210 or P288 cells treated with methotrexate, suggesting that they may be a specific reaction of a particular cell type in response to methotrexate exposure. The particular cell type might be a thymus-derived lymphocyte, since both Sézary cells and CCRF-CEM cells have T cell markers (30, 35).

The molecular basis for methotrexate's nuclear effect was not studied beyond one experiment, in which it was found that the effect was prevented by treatment in 5 μM thymidine and 32 μM hypoxanthine, but not 5 μM thymidine alone. Thus it is related to the known ability of the

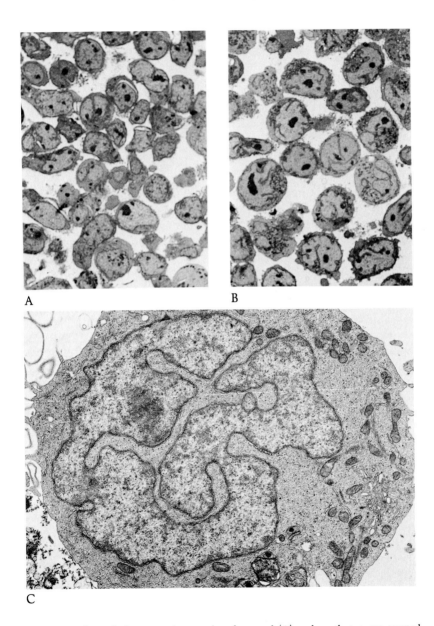

Fig. 9.9 Light and electron micrographs of control (A) and methotrexate-treated (B, C) CCRF-CEM cells. Treatment was in vitro with 10^{-8}M methotrexate for 48 hr. The nuclei of treated cells (B, C) contain numerous indentations of the nuclear envelope, while the control cells (A) do not. Note that the mitochondria are not affected by the drug treatment (C) (A × 975; B × 975; C × 6,000).

drug to perturb purine metabolism (28, 29). Of more significance to the original intention of this study was the finding that the mitochondria were not generally swollen by the drug, even in cells where the nuclear effect was most prominent. Thus the mitochondrial damage observed following treatment with MGBG is drug-specific and not a general phenomenon associated with drug-induced cell death.

Resemblance of Mitochondrial Effect to That Produced by Ethidium Bromide (EB)

The similarity of mitochondrial granule formation by MGBG and EB raises the interesting possibility that the two drugs act by the same molecular mechanism. In fact, the overall mitochondrial damage resulting from the two drugs is quite similar. Like MGBG, EB has been observed to cause selective mitochondrial swelling in L cells (36, 37). A similar swelling has also been observed with chloramphenicol (36), but this drug is not as selective in its effect and tends also to involve the endoplasmic reticulum. The specific effects of EB and MGBG on cell ultrastructure were studied in the same cell line to compare their effects qualitatively and quantitatively. In L1210 cells, the two drugs caused similar mitochondrial damage. Cells treated with EB were enlarged and contained swollen mitochondria with distorted, often tubular, cristae and an electron-lucent matrix (fig. 9.10). Several of the mitochondria contained electron-dense granules similar to those seen in NALM-1 cells. In addition, EB treatment caused a condensation of the nuclear chromatin of L1210 cells and, in that regard, was not as selective in its ultrastructural effects as MGBG. It is interesting that qualitatively similar drug damage to mitochondria could be obtained at approximately the same drug concentrations (EB, $5 \mu M$; MGBG, $10 \mu M$). The EB damage, however, required 48 hr to be qualitatively similar to that produced by MGBG after 24 hr.

The resemblance in structural damage caused by the two drugs and the similarity of both molecules to spermidine (38, 39) increases the possibility that they have a similar molecular action in the mitochondrion. The damage produced by EB is believed to be due to the intercalation of the drug between the base pairs of mitochondrial DNA and to the subsequent inhibition of replication and transcription of genomes (40). Although MGBG binds only weakly to nuclear DNA (41), its ability to interact with the circular mitochondria has not yet been investigated. Recently, MGBG at growth-inhibitory concentrations was found to inhibit incorporation of [³H]-thymidine into mitochondrial DNA (42, 43). After five hours of treatment, this effect was selective for mitochondrial DNA and it preceded the appearance of detectable ultrastructural damage to the mitochondria by several hours. When compared to EB, however, the MGBG effect on mitochondrial DNA was not nearly as remarkable, especially with respect to the impact of the drug on the synthesis of mature circular forms of mitochondrial DNA.

Dependence of Mitochondrial Damage on Cell Proliferation

In the course of examining the generality of MGBG-mitochondrial action in a variety of cell types, it was noted that the onset of visible ultrastructural damage seemed to correlate with generation time. That is, the longer the generation time, the more time required for the ultrastructural damage to occur. Thus mitochondrial damage appeared in L1210 cells (generation time 12 hr) after 12 hr, while qualitatively similar damage was not apparent in NALM-1 cells (generation time 96 hr) until 72 hr. This finding led to the conclusion that the mitochondrial damage might be dependent on cell division. This was tested in two separate culture systems of dividing and nondividing cell populations. In cultures of human peripheral blood lymphocytes stimulated to divide with PHA, only the mitochondria of cells undergoing blastogenesis were damaged by MGBG (fig. 9.11). Other cells present in the culture, including nondividing lymphocytes and macrophages (fig. 9.11), appeared unaffected even when treated for considerably longer periods. Likewise, all lymphoctyes in cultures without PHA were not affected by MGBG.

In the second system, confluent and subconfluent C3H/10T½ mouse embryo fibroblasts (8) were exposed to MGBG. The mitochondria of the subconfluent, but not the confluent, cells were swollen following drug treatment. C3H/10T½ cells are exquisitely sensitive to contact inhibition and cease dividing at confluency (8). Thus only the mitochondria of the dividing subconfluent cells were damaged by MGBG. Results from both systems confirm that cell proliferation is required in order for the drug-induced damage to be expressed. Whether this is related to drug uptake or to mitochondrial biogenesis has not yet been determined. The finding, however, is consistent with the increased levels of polyamines in most proliferating tissues and with the possibility that the mitochondrial damage might be the consequence of inhibition of spermidine and spermine biosynthesis by MGBG. It is interesting, too, that the finding is consistent with the primary toxicity of the drug, which involves proliferating tissues (i.e., marrow, intestine, spleen) and that this toxicity can be reversed by the administration of spermidine (44, 45).

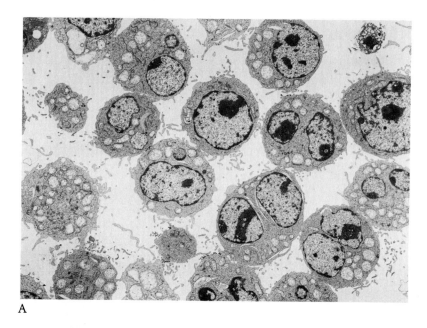

A

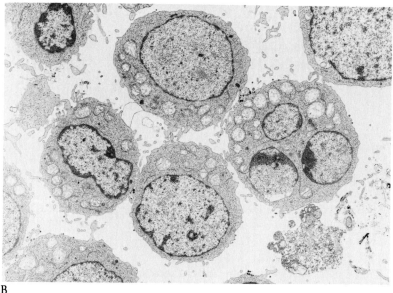

B

Fig. 9.10 L1210 cells treated in culture with 5 μMEB for 24–48 hr. After 48 hr (A, B) the mitochondria of all the cells are swollen, and electron-lucent, and the cristae are vesicular. The chromatin is condensed and stains heavily with uranyl salts. The cristae of mitochondria in cells treated for 24 hr (C) are at first tubular and

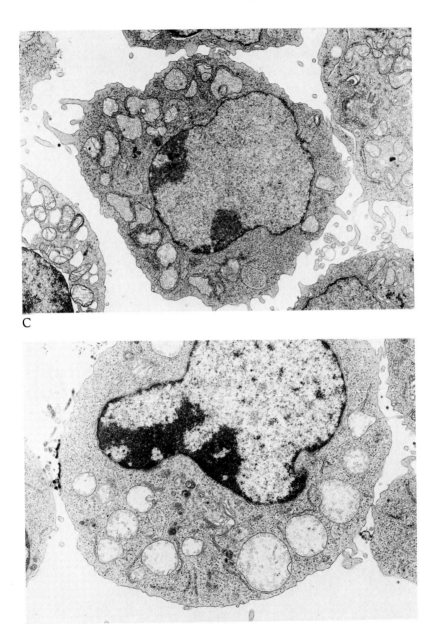

C

D

then by 48 hr (D) appear as tiny vesicles at the internal periphery of the swollen mitochondria. The overall drug effect on the cristae is different from that seen with MGBG (fig. 9.3–9.6) (A × 3,200; B × 3,900; C × 5,900; D × 10,500).

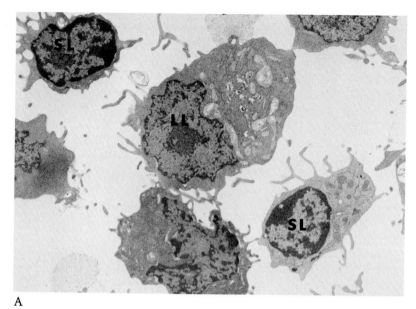

A

B

Fig. 9.11 Phytohemagglutinin (PHA-stimulated cultures of human peripheral blood lymphocytes treated 48 hr with 10 μM MGBG. The mitochondria of large lymphocytes (LL) are swollen, while those of small lymphocytes (A, SL) or macrophages (B, M) are not (A × 4,000; B × 4,000).

Relation of Polyamines to Mitochondrial Damage

It is reasonable to assume that the mitochondrial damage elicited by MGBG might be directly related to antiproliferative activity or, more interestingly, both actions might be consequential to drug interference with polyamine metabolism. In fact, several lines of evidence suggest that the antiproliferative action of MGBG might very well be related to spermidine metabolism or function. These include the following:

1. The effects of MGBG on L1210 leukemia in mice can be prevented by concurrent administration of spermidine (9), spermine, or putrescine (9, 46).
2. There exist basic structural similarities between MGBG and spermidine (47) (fig. 9.2).
3. MGBG and spermidine compete for a common uptake carrier system (48, 49).
4. As noted earlier, MGBG inhibits putrescine-activated S-adenosyl-methionine decarboxylase and hence spermidine and spermine synthesis (13, 14).

On the basis of these data, a number of studies have sought to establish that the antiproliferative effects of MGBG are related to an interference with polyamine metabolism. None have succeeded in doing so, however (12, 15, 16, 17). The fact that the drug has now been shown to have three distinct pharmacological actions (mitochondrial damage included) makes studies relating one drug effect to another even more difficult.

As one approach to this problem, comparative studies of the ultrastructural effects of four drugs, including MGBG, were undertaken. α-Methyl-ornithine and α-difluoromethyl-ornithine (a gift from Centre de Recherche Merrell International, Strasbourg, France) are competitive (50) and irreversible inhibitors (51) respectively of ornithine decarboxylase and have been shown to inhibit polyamine synthesis and cell proliferation in a variety of cultured cells (16, 51, 52, 53). The effects of these drugs were compared ultrastructurally with those of MGBG and 4, 4'-diacetyl-diphenylurea bis(guanylhydrazone) (DDUG). Unlike MGBG, DDUG is an aromatic bis(guanylhydrazone) and has no direct effect on the biosynthesis of polyamines (13). The potent antiproliferative activity of the drug (54, 55) is believed to be due to a primary inhibition of DNA biosynthesis attributed to its ability to bind DNA and inhibit DNA polymerase (41).

α-Methyl-ornithine and α-difluoromethyl-ornithine required millimolar concentrations to attain growth-inhibition kinetics similar to those of 10 μM MGBG. At concentrations up to 50 mM, neither drug had an effect on the ultrastructure of mitochondria or other cellular organelles. DDUG inhibited cell growth at concentrations similar to MGBG and caused distinctive ultrastructural damage to mitochondria. In contrast to the results of MGBG treatment, the mitochondria did not swell as a consequence of DDUG treatment, but became externally lamellated with layers of membranes and contained internal membranous whorls (fig. 9.12). After 24-hr treatment with 5 μM DDUG, most mitochondria of cells were similarly affected, while other organelles appeared normal. The membranous enveloping of mitochondria resembled autophagocytosis in appearance and, in fact, was found cytochemically to have acid phosphatase activity associated with it.

The results obtained with the ornithine decarboxylase inhibitors were equivocal with respect to whether drug perturbation of polyamines leads to mitochondrial damage. The lack of effect with these drugs suggests that it does not. The concentrations of MGBG required to produce mitochondrial damage decrease intracellular spermidine pools to levels that are still above those after treatment with α-methyl-ornithine (45). But while MGBG causes a decrease in intracellular spermidine pools, it also causes a marked increase in putrescine pools which α-methyl-ornithine and α-difluoromethyl-ornithine do not (16, 51, 52, 53). Therefore, the effects of these drugs on polyamines may not be immediately comparable and this may

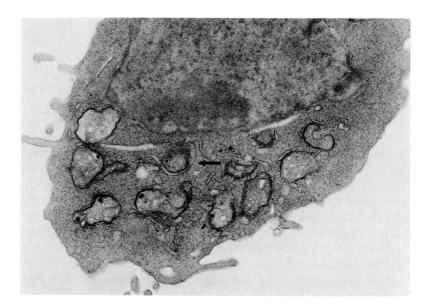

Fig. 9.12 Cytoplasm of an L1210 cell treated 24 hr with 5 μM 4,4'-diacetyldiphenylurea bis(guanylhydrazone) (DDUG). The mitochondria are enveloped in layers of myelinlike membrane that appears to be derived from endoplasmic reticulum (arrow). At this point the cristae are still visible inside (× 10,500).

account for the lack of mitochondrial damage done by the ornithine analogs.

Results with DDUG are equally as uninformative with regard to polyamine involvement in MGBG-induced mitochondrial damage. The DDUG lesion, although selective for mitochondria, was clearly distinct from that seen with MGBG and therefore exempt from direct correlations. The lesion itself closely resembled the ultrastructural events associated with autophagocytosis (56). Whorls of endoplasmic reticulum enwrapped mitochondria. When the enclosure of myelin-type membranes was complete, the internal cristae of the mitochondria dissolved away, leaving an amorphous interior. Thus the cell may attempt to remove drug-damaged mitochondria by this mechanism, as is known to be the case in hepatocytes exposed to glucagon (57), in mice mammary tumors treated with cyclophosphamide (58), or in fibrosarcoma cells treated with thio-TEPA (59). Whether cells treated with DDUG can then repopulate their cytoplasm with new mitochondria and recover normal growth characteristics was not examined.

The different ultrastructural appearance of mitochondria exposed to DDUG or MGBG may be related to the physical properties of the two drugs. DDUG has been found to have a strong affinity for phospholipids, excepting those containing a choline molecule, while MGBG does not (60). Another antineoplastic agent, acronycin, causes swelling and destruction of the Golgi complexes and, less consistently, swelling of mitochondria (61). The general action by acronycin involving membranous organelles is thought to be due to the lipophilic nature of the drug. In the case of DDUG, however, the ultrastructural damage is specific for mitochondria, and the Golgi region is unaffected by the drug so that the drug effect is not entirely attributable to its lipophilic nature.

Although DDUG has potent activity against in vitro test systems, no therapeutic effect was seen in initial clinical studies (45). The results from the present study suggest that it may have usefulness as an experimental tool for the study of mitochondrial biogenesis or autophagocytosis.

Mitochondrial Damage with In Vivo MGBG or EB Treatment and Its Reversibility

In order to establish that the mitochondrial damage produced in cultured cells by MGBG may, in fact, account for or contribute to the clinical activity of the drug, mice bearing L1210 leukemia were treated in vivo with MGBG and the cells examined ultrastructurally for mitochondrial damage. For comparison purposes, mice were also treated with EB and similarly examined. At concentrations of MGBG regarded as

pharmacological (50 mg/kg, single I.P. injection), the mitochondria of
L1210 cells taken 24 hr after drug injection appeared much the same as in
MGBG-treated cultured cells (62). Although not distended quite so extensively as with in vitro drug treatment, the mitochondria were nonetheless
distinctly swollen and exhibited the same loss of cristae and matrix. In the
case of EB-treated cells examined 24 hr after a single 50 mg/kg I.P.
injection, the mitochondria were also swollen but, in addition, frequently
contained a flocculent electron density (fig. 9.8) which is consistent with
findings for cells treated with EB in culture (23, 24). It is interesting to
again note the similarities in dosages for EB and MGBG that were required
to elicit the mitochondrial damage.

Inhibition of respiration and energy production have been demonstrated
to be important factors in eliciting mitochondrial damage. Studies by Laiho
and Trump (63) suggest that the occurrence of swelling indicates structural
changes in the mitochondrial inner membrane following loss of ability for
adenosine 5'-triphosphate (ATP) synthesis. High-pressure liquid chromatographic analyses of the ribonucleotide pools of cells treated with
either MGBG or EB are markedly depleted, especially the ATP pools (62).
As a consequence, the overall adenylate charge of the cell decreases from
about 0.8 for control cells to about 0.5 for EB- or MGBG-treated cells. The
results demonstrate that the structurally damaged mitochondria are indeed
functionally impaired as well and to such an extent that other cellular
phenomena could be affected. The results corroborate findings by Pine and
DiPaolo (21), who reported that cellular respiration was partly inhibited by
MGBG and that phosphorylation of isolated mitochondria was uncoupled.

The reversibility of the structural and functional lesion induced in
mitochondria by either MGBG or EB was tested by taking ascites cells
treated in vivo as just described and reinjecting them into the abdomen of
another untreated mouse. After 24 hr under these recovery conditions, the
mitochondria of cells initially treated with MGBG were still swollen but
not as much as immediately after drug treatment. By the 48th hr of
recovery, the mitochondria were no longer swollen and appeared similar to
those of control cells. Structural recovery was accompanied by a recovery
of functional capabilities, as indicated by the increase in intracellular ATP
pools and a concomitant increase in the adenylate energy charge to levels
of control cells (about 0.8). Thus despite the extent of the original
ultrastructural damage, the MGBG-treated cells were able to reverse the
drug effect when grown in the absence of the drug. The morphology of the
reversal suggests that it is accomplished by repair and restoration of
damaged mitochondria rather than replacement with new organelles, as
has been observed in cultured cells treated with EB (37, 64).

Neither morphologic nor functional recovery of cells treated with EB was achieved in the absence of the drug (62). Even after 72 hr in the untreated mouse, the mitochondria still appeared damaged. While most of the mitochondria were swollen, some appeared small and condensed, suggesting that repopulation by new mitochondria might be taking place, as has been observed to occur in cultured L cells treated with EB (37).

Overall, the in vivo studies have demonstrated that 1) MGBG mitochondrial damage occurs in cells treated in vivo as well as in culture; 2) the mitochondria are functionally compromised by the drug; 3) under the present conditions of MGBG treatment, the lesion is sublethal and reversible; and 4) the mitochondrial damage produced under present experimental conditions by EB in ascites L1210 cells is not reversible. Whether the structural damage produced by MGBG precedes the functional impairment or the opposite occurs was not investigated but could provide insight into cause and effect, especially if carefully correlated with fluctuations in intracellular adenosine pools.

Basis for the MGBG Mitochondrial Damage and Its Relevance to Inhibition of Cell Proliferation

At present, the molecular basis for the selective ultrastructural damage to mitochondria by MGBG is unknown. In one recent study (42, 43), it was found that treatment of L1210 cells in vitro with MGBG at concentrations of greater than 1 μM results in inhibition of mitochondrial DNA synthesis but not nuclear DNA synthesis at treatment times up to 5 hr. The earliest detectable effect on mitochondrial DNA with 10 μM MGBG occurs at 1.5 hr, which is well before the first ultrastructural damage for L1210 spinner cultures (6 hr); and the minimum MGBG concentration which causes ultrastructural damage and interference with mitochondrial DNA is the same, 1 μM. This suggests that a cause and effect relationship may exist for the two drug actions, but it is possible that both are secondary to a singular action of the drug on another aspect of cell metabolism, possibly involving the polyamines.

Since mitochondrial damage has consistently been found to precede drug inhibition of cell growth by several hours, it is tempting to speculate that the mitochondrial lesion is, in fact, responsible for growth inhibition. This idea is further reinforced by the finding that mitochondrial damage only appears in proliferating cells. Yet there is little evidence in the literature to indicate that cells are so dependent on their mitochondria, especially cells in culture, which are known to rely heavily on glycolysis for ATP production. Recent studies with EB (65) indicate that when the ATP of mitochondria of yeast is depleted by use of an inhibitor of mitochondrial adenine nucleotide translocation system together with EB, the cells lose their ability to proliferate. This occurs despite the fact that ATP is adequately generated by glycolysis. The authors conclude that the mitochondrion has a direct or indirect role in the control of cell proliferation. It remains conceivable, therefore, that inhibition of cell growth by MGBG is a consequence of drug action on mitochondria. If confirmed, the potential of this organelle as a target for cancer chemotherapy should be reevaluated.

Concluding Remarks

The anticancer agent, MGBG, and certain structurally or functionally related drugs have been used as examples to illustrate how ultrastructural studies can serve alone or in conjunction with biochemical studies to investigate the mode of action of drugs. Unquestionably, such studies are only feasible when the drug examined produces a unique structural lesion that can be clearly distinguished from nonspecific changes associated with cell death. Although such lesions are often regarded as exceptional, our experience, as shown here by several examples, indicates that given the appropriate conditions they are a fairly common phenomenon which could be exploited more in the study of drug action.

In the case of MGBG in particular, ultrastructural studies have generated new and interesting information of pharmacological relevance. These studies have served to rekindle the significance of the previously noted antimitochondrial action of the drug. Much of the current dogma regarding MGBG tends to attribute its antiproliferative action to interference with polyamine metabolism despite the fact that the essentiality of these molecules in dividing cell populations has never been established. In fact, the antiproliferative action of MGBG has often been cited as evidence for the latter.

From the ultrastructural data obtained from a variety of systems, the general impression gained is that the action of MGBG on mitochondria may be responsible for the growth-inhibitory effect and deserves further consideration. The intriguing possibility of biological interest that must be considered is that the polyamines are in some way essential to the structure and/or function of mitochondria. Alternatively, the drug may act directly on some critical mitochondrial component (i.e., the cytochromes) in addition to perturbing polyamine metabolism.

In view of the outstanding toxicity that accompanies the neoplastic action of MGBG in animals and in human beings, it is important that the basis for this toxicity be clarified. Of primary interest is the determination of the extent to which the drug-induced mitochondrial damage contributes to host toxicity, and an exploration of means by which this action can be minimized while still preserving the antineoplastic action of the drug. In short, the selectivity of the drug must be improved. This could involve administration of certain agents such as spermidine either during or following MGBG treatment in an attempt to protect or rescue host tissues respectively. Alternatively, in view of the significance of the mito-chondrial action of the drug, new drug combinations, possibly using an inhibitor of glycolysis, could be devised to avoid host toxicity by either drug. Such innovations may increase the therapeutic advantages of MGBG by increasing the selectivity of the antineoplastic action, and their success in achieving this goal could be continually monitored by ultrastructural studies in which the mitochondrial lesion would serve as a sensitive indicator for host toxicity.

References

1. Di Marco, A. Adriamycin (NSC-123127), mode and mechanism of action. *Cancer Treat. Rep.* Part 3, 6(2):91–106, 1975.

2. Smetana, K. et al. Effect of adriamycin on nucleolar morphology: a simple biologic assay. *Cancer Treat. Rep.* 61:1253–1259, 1977.

3. Simond, R. The nucleus: action of chemical and physical agents. *Int. Rev. Cytol.* 28:169–211, 1970.

4. Herman, L., and Fitzgerald, P. The degenerative changes in pancreatic acinar cells caused by DL-ethionine. *J. Cell Biol.* 12:277, 1962.

5. Sinozuka, M. P.; Goldblatt, P. J.; and Farber, E. The disorganization of hepatic cell nucleoli induced by ethionine and its reversal by adenine. *J. Cell Biol.* 36:313, 1968.

6. Chevremont, M.; Chevremont-Combaire, S.; and Firket, H. Study of the action of ribonuclease on living cells cultivated *in vitro* and in particular of the effects on mitosis. *Arch. Biol.* (Liege) 65:635–656, 1956.

7. Minowada, J. et al. A non-T, non-B human leukemia cell line (NALM-1): establishment of the cell line and presence of leukemia-associated antigens. *JNCI* 59:83–97, 1977.

8. Reznikoff, C. A. et al. Quantitative and qualitative studies of chemical transformation of cloned C3H mouse embryo cells sensitive to postconfluence inhibition of cell division. *Cancer Res.* 33:3239–3249, 1973.

9. Mihich, E. Current studies with methylglyoxal-bis(guanylhydrazone). *Cancer Res.* 23:1375–1389, 1963.

10. Levin, R. H. et al. Treatment of acute leukemia with methylglyoxal-bis-guanylhydrazone (methyl GAG). *Clin. Pharmacol. Ther.* 6:31–42, 1964.

11. Knight, W. A. et al. Methylglyoxal-bis(guanylhydrazone) (methyl GAG, MGBG) in advanced human malignancy. *Proc. Am. Assoc. Cancer Res.* 20:319, 1979.

12. Dave, C.; Ehrke, J. M.; and Mihich, E. Studies on the structure activity relationship among aliphatic and aromatic bis-(guanylhydrazones) and some related compounds. *Chem. Biol. Interact.* 16:57–68, 1977.

13. Corti, A. et al. Specific inhibition of the enzyme decarboxylation of S-adenosylmethionine by methylglyoxal-bis(guanylhydrazone) and related substances. *Biochem. J.* 139:351–357, 1974.

14. Williams-Ashman, H. G., and Shenone, A. Methylglyoxal-bis-(guanylhydrazone) as a potent inhibitor of mammalian and yeast S-adenosyl-methionine decarboxylases. *Biochem. Biophys. Res. Commun.* 46:288–295, 1972.

15. Fillingame, R. H.; Jorstad, C. M.; and Morris, D. R. Increased cellular levels of spermidine or spermine are required for optimal DNA synthesis in lymphocytes activated by concanavalin A. *Proc. Natl. Acad. Sci. USA* 72:4042–4045, 1975.

16. Morris, D. R.; Jorstad, C. M.; and Seyfried, C. E. Inhibition of the synthesis of polyamines and DNA in activated lymphocytes by a combination of α-methyl-ornithine and methylglyoxal-bis(guanylhydrazone). *Cancer Res.* 37:3169–3172, 1977.

17. Otani, S. et al. Inhibition of DNA synthesis by methylglyoxal-bis-(guanylhydrazone) during lymphocyte transformation. *Mol. Biol. Rep.* 1:431–436, 1974.

18. Brown, K. B.; Nelson, N. F.; and Brown, D. G. Effects of polyamines and methylglyoxal-bis(guanylhydrazone) on hepatic nuclear structure and deoxyribo-nucleic acid template activity. *Biochem. J.* 151:505–512, 1975.

19. Gfeller, E. et al. Ultrastructural changes *in vitro* of rat liver nucleoli in response to polyamines. *Z. Zellforsch.* 129:447–454, 1972.

20. Pathak, S. N.; Porter, C. W.; and Dave, C. Morphological evidence for antimitochondrial action by methylglyoxal-bis(guanylhydrazone). *Cancer Res.* 37:2246–2250, 1977.

21. Pine, M. J., and Di Paolo, J. A. The antimitochondrial action of 2-chloro-4′,4″-bis(2-imidazolin-2-yl)terephthalanilide and methylglyoxal-bis-(guanylhydrazone). *Cancer Res.* 26:18–25, 1966.

22. Peachy, L. D. Electron microscope observations on the accumulation of divalent cations in intramitochondrial granules. *J. Cell Biol.* 20:95–111, 1964.

23. McGill, M.; Hsu, T. C.; and Brinkley, B. R. Electron-dense structures in mitochondria induced by short-term ethidium bromide treatment. *J. Cell Biol.* 59:260–265, 1973.

24. McGill, M.; Baur, P. S.; and Hsu, T. C. Ultrastructural and microchemical composition of ethidium bromide-induced intramitochondrial complexes. *Exp. Cell Res.* 99:7–14, 1976.

25. Saladino, A. J.; Bentley, P. J.; and Trump, B. F. Ion movements in cell injury. Effect of amphotericin B on the ultrastructure and function of the epithelial cells of the toad bladder. *Am. J. Pathol.* 54:421, 1969.

26. Trump, B. F., and Ericsson, J. E. L. Some ultrastructural and biochemical consequences of cell injury. P. 35 in *The inflammatory process*, ed. B. W. Zweifach, L. Grant, and L. McCluskey. New York: Academic Press, Inc., 1965.

27. Foley, G. E. et al. Continuous culture of human lymphoblasts from peripheral blood of a child with acute leukemia. *Cancer* 18:522–529, 1965.

28. Bertino, F. The mechanism of action of the folate antagonists in man. *Cancer Res.* 23:1286–1291, 1963.

29. Werkheiser, W. The biochemical, cellular and pharmacological action and effects of the folic acid antagonists. *Cancer Res.* 23:1277–1285, 1963.

30. Lutzner, M. A.; Hobbs, J. W.; and Horvath, P. Ultrastructure of abnormal cells in Sézary's syndrome, mycosis fungoides, and parapsoriasis in plaque. *Arch. Dermatol.* 103:375–386, 1971.

31. Smith, H. S.; Springer, C. L.; and Hackett, A. J. Nuclear ultrastructure of epithelial cell lines derived from human carcinomas and nonmalignant tissues. *Cancer Res.* 39:332–344, 1979.

32. Biberfeld, P. Morphogenesis of blood lymphocytes stimulated with phytohaemagglutinin (PHA)—a light and electron microscope study. *Acta Pathol. Microbiol. Scand.* (Suppl. A) 223:1–70, 1971.

33. Horvath, E.; Kovacs, K.; and Roos, R. C. Liver ultrastructure in methotrexate treatment of psoriasis. *Arch. Dermatol.* 108:427–428, 1973.

34. Nyfors, A., and Hopwood, D. Liver ultrastructure in psoriatives related to methotrexate therapy. *Acta. Pathol. Microbiol. Scand.* [A] 85:787–800, 1977.

35. Minowada, J. et al. Expression of an antigen associated with acute lymphoblastic leukemia in human leukemia-lymphoma cell lines. *JNCI* 60:1269–1276, 1978.

36. King, M. E.; Godman, G. C.; and King, D. W. Respiratory enzymes and mitochondrial morphology of HeLa and L cells treated with chloramphenicol and ethidium bromide. *J. Cell Biol.* 53:127–142, 1972.

37. Soslau, G., and Naas, M. M. K. Effects of ethidium bromide on the cytochrome content and ultrastructure of L cell mitochondria. *J. Cell Biol.* 51:514–525, 1971.

38. Cohen, S. S. What do the polyamines do? *Nature* 247:209–210, 1978.

39. Williams-Ashman, H. G.; Corti, A.; and Tadolini, B. On the development of specific inhibitors of animal polyamine biosynthetic enzymes. *Ital. J. Biochem.* 25:5–32, 1977.

40. Waring, M. J. Drugs which affect the structure and function of DNA. *Nature* 219:1320–1322, 1968.

41. Dave, C.; Ehrke, J.; and Mihich, E. Spectrophotometric studies on the binding with polynucleotides of 4,4'-diacetyldiphenylurea-bis(guanylhydrazone) and methylglyoxal-bis(guanylhydrazone). *Chem. Biol. Interact.* 12:183–195, 1976.

42. Feuerstein, B.; Porter, C. W.; and Dave, C. Comparative effects of methylglyoxal-bis(guanylhydrazone) (MGBG) on mitochrondrial (mt) and nuclear (n) DNA of mouse leukemia L-1210 cells in culture. *Fed. Proc.* 37:900, 1978.

43. Feuerstein, B; Porter, C. W.; and Dave, C. A selective effect of methylglyoxal-bis(guanylhydrazone) on the mitochondrial DNA of L-1210 cells in culture. *Cancer Res.* 39:4130–4137, 1979.

44. Mihich, E. Impairment of host defenses by methylglyoxal-bis-(guanylhydrazone). *Fed. Proc.* 23:388, 1964.

45. Mihich, E. Bis-guanylhydrazones. Pp. 766–788 in *Handbook of experimental pharmacology*, vol. 38, ed. A. C. Sartorelli and D. G.Johns. New York: Springer-Verlag New York, Inc., 1975.

46. Mihich, E. Prevention of the antitumor activity of methylglyoxal-bis(guanylhydrazone) (CH_3-G) by spermidine. *Pharmacologist* 5:270, 1963.

47. Hamilton, W. C., and Laplaca, S. J. The crystal and molecular structure of antileukemic drug methylglyoxal-bis(guanylhydrazone) dihydrochloride monohydrate, $C_5N_3H_{12} \cdot 2HCl \cdot H_2O$ neutron and x-ray diffraction studies. *Acta Cryst.* B24:1147–1156, 1968.

48. Field, M. et al. Cellular accumulation of methylglyoxal-bis-(guanylhydrazone) in vitro. I. General characteristics of cellular uptake. *Cancer Res.* 24:1939–1946, 1964.

49. Dave, C., and Caballes, L. Studies on the uptake of methylglyoxal-bis(guanylhydrazone) (CH_3G) and Spermidine (spd) in mouse leukemia L-1210 sensitive and resistant to CH_3G (L-1210/CH_3G). *Fed. Proc.* 32:736, 1973.

50. Abdel-Monem, M. M.; Newton, N. E.; and Weeks, C. E. Inhibitors of polyamine biosynthesis. I. α-methyl-($\pm$)-ornithine, an inhibitor of ornithine decarboxylase. *J. Med. Chem.* 17:447–451, 1974.

51. Mamont, P. S. et al. Antiproliferative properties of DL-α-fluoromethyl ornithine in cultured cells. A consequence of the irreversible inhibition of ornithine decarboxylase. *Biochem. Biophys. Res. Commun.* 81:58–66, 1978.

52. Mamont, P. S. et al. α-methylornithine, a potent competitive inhibitor of ornithine decarboxylase, blocks proliferation of rat hepatoma cells in culture. *Proc. Natl. Acad. Sci. USA* 73:1626–1630, 1976.

53. Newton, N. E., and Abdel-Monem, M. M. Inhibitors of polyamine bio-synthesis. 4. Effects of α-methyl-($\pm$)-ornithine and methylglyoxal-bis(guanyl-hydrazone) on growth and polyamine content of L-1210 leukemic cells of mice. *J. Med. Chem.* 20:249–253, 1977.

54. Mihich, E., and Gelzer, J. Effects of 4,4'-diacetyl-diphenyl-urea-bis-(guanylhydrazone) on a spectrum of mouse and rat tumors. *Cancer Res.* 28:553–558, 1968.

55. Mihich, E., and Mulhern, A. I. Effects of 4,4'-diacetyl-diphenyl-urea-bis(guanylhydrazone) on a leukemia L-1210. *Cancer Res.* 28:354–362, 1968.

56. Ericsson, J. L. W. Mechanism of cellular autophagy. Pp. 345–394 in *Lysosomes in biology and pathology*, vol. 2, ed. J. T. Dingle and H. B. Fell. New York: American Elsevier Publishers, Inc., 1970.

57. Deter, R. L.; Baudhuin, P.; and DeDuve, C. Participation of lysosomes in cellular autophage induced in rat liver by glucagon. *J. Cell Biol.* 35:C11, 1967.

58. Anton, E., and Brandes, D. Lysosomes in mice mammary tumors treated with cyclophosphamide. *Cancer* 21:483–500, 1968.

59. Barton, A. A., and Barton, M. The function of membranes in neoplastic cells partially resistant to thiotepa. *Int. J. Cancer* 3:137–141, 1968.

60. Hakala, M. T. Uptake and distribution of 4,4'-diacetyl-diphenyl-urea-bis-(guanylhydrazone) in sensitive and resistant sarcoma 180 cells *in vitro. Biochem. Pharmacol.* 20:81–95, 1971.

61. Tan, P., and Auersperg, N. Effects of the antineoplastic alkaloid acronycin on the ultrastructure and growth patterns of cultured cells. *Cancer Res.* 33:2320–2329, 1973.

62. Porter, C. W. et al. Correlation of ultrastructural and functional damage to mitochondria of ascites L-1210 cells treated *in vivo* with methylglyoxal-

bis(guanylhydrazone) (MGBG) or ethidium bromide (EB). *Cancer Res.* 39:2414–2421, 1979.

63. Laiho, K. V., and Trump, B. F. Studies on the pathogenesis of cell injury. Effects of inhibitors of metabolism and membrane function on mitochondria of Ehrlich ascites tumor cells. *Lab. Invest.* 32:163–182, 1965.

64. Koblinsky, L., and Beattie, D. S. The reversibility of the ethidium bromide-induced alterations of mitochondrial structure and function in the cellular slime mold, *Dictyostelium discoideum. J. Bionerg. Biomembr.* 9:73–90, 1977.

65. Kovac, L.; Kolarov, J.; and Subik, J. Genetic determination of the mitochondrial adenine nucleotide translocation system and its role in the eukaryotic cell. *Mol. Cell. Biochem.* 14:11–14, 1977.

Index

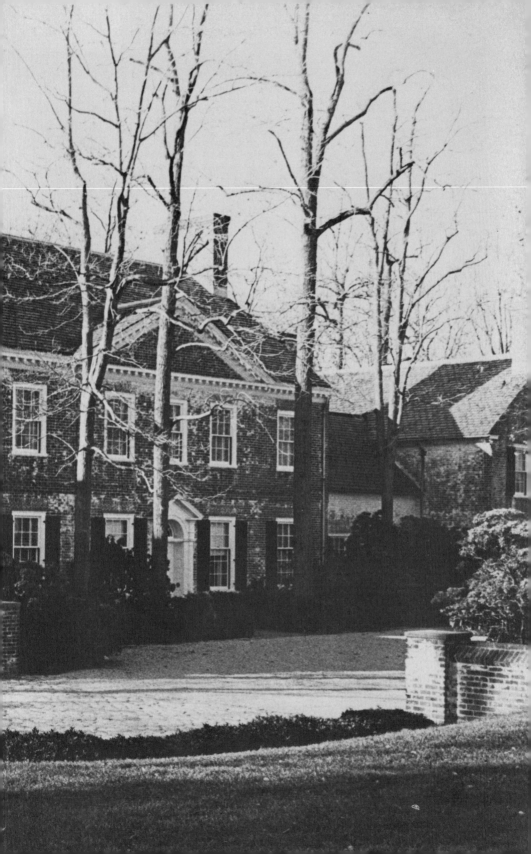